P[illegible]

WHAT'S MAKING OUR CHILDREN SICK?

"Through surveys, doctors' reports, and countless firsthand discussions, we are aware that thousands of people get better from a wide range of diseases and conditions soon after switching to a non-GMO organic diet. This outstanding book not only sees the results every day in Dr. Perro's practice, but has also connected the dots with the science. *What's Making Our Children Sick?* should be required reading for every doctor, every mom, and anyone seeking to prevent or reverse a chronic condition."

—**Jeffrey M. Smith**, author of *Seeds of Deception* and *Genetic Roulette*; codirector of *Secret Ingredients*

"It would be difficult for anyone to read this powerful book with even a halfway open mind and not conclude that our industrialized system of food production is in urgent need of major reform. The routine claim that genetically engineered foods are well-regulated, well-tested, and wholesome crumples in the face of the facts that are skillfully woven together in this monumental work."

—**Steven M. Druker**, author of *Altered Genes, Twisted Truth: How the Venture to Genetically Engineer Our Food Has Subverted Science, Corrupted Government, and Systematically Deceived the Public*

"Chronic diseases that were once rare are now plaguing children and adults alike in industrialized nations such as the United States. The patient case histories that Dr. Perro and Dr. Adams describe in *What's Making Our Children Sick?* provide compelling evidence for advocating lifestyle changes, especially dietary medicine intervention, for overcoming these chronic ailments. And science increasingly provides explanations for such success. We now know that the balance of our gut bacteria (microbiome) is crucial to health and that imbalance, causing gut dysbiosis, is at least a contributing factor to a vast range of chronic illnesses, both physical and mental. Poor diet is no doubt a major contributory factor in causing gut dysbiosis. By eliminating pesticide and GMO-laden food from the diet and replacing it with organic wholefoods as part of her lifestyle medicine approach, Dr. Perro succeeds where standard pharmaceuticals fail. This should be enough for all to take note and follow suit."

—**Michael Antoniou**, molecular geneticist, King's College London; coauthor of *GMO Myths and Truths*

"The sharp rise of severe allergies, brain disorders, and other chronic illnesses among America's children has left many doctors stumped, finding themselves unable to offer lasting cures or even successfully manage sometimes devastating symptoms. Enter Dr. Michelle Perro, an integrative food-forward family physician who has had excellent results helping children and adults overcome chronic disease. Even if you're already familiar with the controversies surrounding genetically modified foods and healthy eating, you will learn a lot from Perro and Adams's carefully researched, science-oriented book. A compelling and important read. Highly recommended."

—**Jennifer Margulis**, PhD, author of *Your Baby, Your Way: Taking Charge of Your Pregnancy, Childbirth, and Parenting Decisions for a Happier, Healthier Family*

"With her extensive experience as a director and attending in Pediatric Emergency Medicine and her current integrative practice and health advocacy, Dr. Michelle Perro has teamed up with coauthor Vincanne Adams, whose expertise from medical anthropology is a perfect complement to the clinical perspective; together they have produced a powerful book. Their analysis carefully examines the scientific evidence and patient responses to the disruptive effects of chemicals contaminating our food, water, and the environment, and their damaging effects on our children. *What's Making Our Children Sick?* exposes the hype of genetic engineering, both its flawed science and failed promises that have wreaked havoc on our health. Using their medical experience and case studies, Perro and Adams offer welcome alternatives to restore our health and hope for our future."

—**Don M. Huber**, emeritus professor, Purdue University

"Having seen firsthand how Dr. Michelle Perro works miracles with children in her clinical practice, I am delighted to see that she has made her insights and approach widely accessible in this groundbreaking book. *What's Making Our Children Sick?* combines the latest research on gut health and the microbiome with concerning evidence about the dangers of genetically modified and industrial foods to elucidate the perfect storm that is damaging our children's health today. Most importantly, it offers practical and actionable solutions for both parents and practitioners to help children recover their health."

—**Akil Palanisamy**, MD, Harvard-trained physician; author of *The Paleovedic Diet*

"Doctors Perro and Adams have made the complex topic of the interrelationship between the gut, brain, and the food our kids eat accessible to all. In my own experience, autism recovery is rarely possible without a dietary overhaul and a focus on whole, organic, and natural foods. This book is a welcome resource for parents struggling with their children's chronic health conditions."

—**J. B. Handley**, cofounder, Generation Rescue

"*What's Making Our Children Sick?* is a true clarion call to parents, physicians, and policymakers everywhere to change the way we grow the food we eat. Unless we move away from industrialized food sources that are created for the lowest short-term costs, we and our children will continue to experience increased chronic disease, immune dysfunction, and mental health problems. The transformation of our nutrition is not simply for our children and us, but also for future generations and our dear planet. It is almost as though we are all Romans drinking wine out of lead-lined bottles. Future generations will wonder why we have been so blind, deaf, and dumb."

—**Dana Ullman**, MPH, CCH, author of *Homeopathic Medicine for Childrenand Infants* and *The Homeopathic Revolution*

"Industrial medicine and agriculture, with wholesale government approval, have caused an epidemic of chronic childhood illness largely traceable to ubiquitous poisons and alien DNA in our food supply. A clinical argument for organic foods, *What's Making Our Children Sick?* is a stop-look-listen book for parents, doctors, teachers, and grocery shoppers everywhere."

—**Carol Van Strum**, author of *A Bitter Fog: Herbicides and Human Rights*

"Dr. Perro was one of the first American pediatricians to connect the dots from GMOs to intestinal permeability, suffering children, and overwhelmed parents. Over the years her knowledge base for solutions has increased exponentially, as has the health of her young patients. Food-focused medicine, as she and Vincanne Adams detail in *What's Making Our Children Sick?*, is a clarion call to us all."

—**Samm Simpson**, cohost, The Power Hour Radio Broadcast; associate producer, *Genetic Roulette*

"Perro and Adams' book is an alarming, eye-opening read that documents more clearly than ever the devastating consequences that pervasive pesticide use in food production is having on our health, and the urgent need to protect our children from a system that prefers we treat illness and disease with pills rather than prevention."

—**Carey Gillam**, journalist, author; research director, consumer advocacy group U.S. Right to Know

"In this important book, pediatrician Michelle Perro and medical anthropologist Vincanne Adams explore Dr. Perro's clinical case histories and the scientific literature to find out what's at the root of the problem. They are convinced that our industrialized food is a chief culprit. Pesticides and genetically modified (GM) foods have introduced known and potential toxins into the food supply, turning it into a "slow poison." Time and again, seemingly intractable health problems in Dr. Perro's young patients respond well, sometimes almost miraculously, when chemically grown and GM foods are eliminated from the diet and replaced with organic foods. No matter how many of the agrichemical industry's lobbyists and PR people bombard us with claims that pesticide residues and GMOs in our foods are safe, the experiences of Dr. Perro's patients are hard to deny and tell a different story. The book is a must-read for health practitioners and parents alike."

—**Claire Robinson**, editor, GMWatch; coauthor of *GMO Myths and Truths*

"Perro and Adams offer a unique analysis regarding the role industrialized food plays in the decline of our children's health. *What's Making our Children Sick?* provides an uncommon but extraordinary blend of clinical medicine and medical anthropology via an expert, in-depth analysis as to the root cause of this health epidemic, beginning with the gut. Filled with both knowledge and compassion, the authors, on a step-by-step readable journey, reveal how our children have become toxic from the very foods that are purportedly nutritious. This book will have wide readership from those who want to improve their own children's health to the medical clinics of healthcare providers."

—**Dr. Richard Horowitz,** bestselling author of *How Can I Get Better? An Action Plan for Treating Resistant Lyme and Chronic Disease*

"A powerful exposé of the science and clinical evidence pointing to our food production system as a key cause of the chronic illnesses affecting so many children. Most importantly, *What's Making Our Children Sick?* offers hope and a path forward for how food-focused medicine can heal our bodies and help our families."

—**Stacy Malkan**, author of *Not Just a Pretty Face: The Ugly Side of the Beauty Industry*

"In a world where we are overexposed to thousands of dangerous toxic chemicals, education is key. This book's clear, comprehensive information is a godsend for parents with sick children, and clinicians in the dark about the cause of the epidemic of chronically ill kids. Bravo to Drs. Perro and Adams for opening our eyes to what's really going on."

—**Beth Greer,** bestselling author of *Super Natural Home*

What's Making Our Children SICK?

What's Making Our Children SICK?

How Industrial Food Is Causing an Epidemic of Chronic Illness, and What Parents (and Doctors) Can Do About It

Michelle Perro, MD *and*
Vincanne Adams, PhD

CHELSEA GREEN PUBLISHING
WHITE RIVER JUNCTION, VERMONT

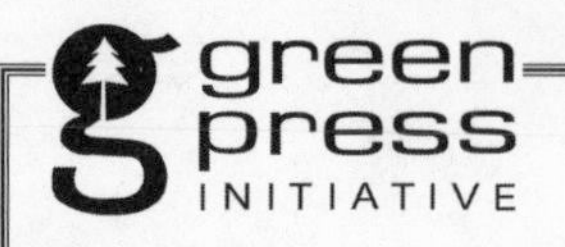

Project Manager: Patricia Stone
Developmental Editor: Makenna Goodman
Copy Editor: Deborah Heimann
Proofreader: Nanette Bendyna
Indexer: Shana Milkie
Designer: Melissa Jacobson

Printed in the United States of America.
First printing November, 2017.
10 9 8 7 6 5 4 3 2 1   17 18 19 20 21

Chelsea Green Publishing is committed to preserving ancient forests and natural resources. We elected to print this title on 100-percent postconsumer recycled paper, processed chlorine-free. As a result, for this printing, we have saved:

60 Trees (40' tall and 6-8" diameter)
27 Million BTUs of Total Energy
5,166 Pounds of Greenhouse Gases
28,019 Gallons of Wastewater
1,876 Pounds of Solid Waste

Chelsea Green Publishing made this paper choice because we and our printer, Thomson-Shore, Inc., are members of the Green Press Initiative, a nonprofit program dedicated to supporting authors, publishers, and suppliers in their efforts to reduce their use of fiber obtained from endangered forests. For more information, visit: www.greenpressinitiative.org.

Environmental impact estimates were made using the Environmental Defense Paper Calculator. For more information visit: www.papercalculator.org.

Our Commitment to Green Publishing

Chelsea Green sees publishing as a tool for cultural change and ecological stewardship. We strive to align our book manufacturing practices with our editorial mission and to reduce the impact of our business enterprise in the environment. We print our books and catalogs on chlorine-free recycled paper, using vegetable-based inks whenever possible. This book might cost slightly more because it was printed on paper that contains recycled fiber, and we hope you'll agree that it's worth it. Chelsea Green is a member of the Green Press Initiative (www.greenpressinitiative.org), a nonprofit coalition of publishers, manufacturers, and authors working to protect the world's endangered forests and conserve natural resources. *What's Making Our Children Sick?* was printed on paper supplied by Thomson-Shore that contains 100% postconsumer recycled fiber.

Library of Congress Cataloging-in-Publication Data
Names: Perro, Michelle, author.
Title: What's making our children sick? : how industrial food is causing an epidemic of chronic illness, and what parents (and doctors) can do about it / Michelle Perro, MD, and Vincanne Adams, PhD.
Description: White River Junction, Vermont : Chelsea Green Publishing, [2017] | Includes bibliographical references and index.
Identifiers: LCCN 2017033470| ISBN 9781603587570 (paperback) | ISBN 9781603587587 (ebook)
Subjects: LCSH: Chronically ill children—Nutrition—Popular works. | Food industry and trade—Health aspects. —Popular works. | Genetically modified foods—Health aspects—Popular works. | Child rearing—Health aspects. | BISAC: HEALTH & FITNESS / Nutrition. | FAMILY & RELATIONSHIPS / Parenting / General. | TECHNOLOGY & ENGINEERING / Food Science. | MEDICAL / Toxicology.
Classification: LCC RJ380 .P48 2017 | DDC 362.19892—dc23
LC record available at https://lccn.loc.gov/2017033470

Chelsea Green Publishing
85 North Main Street, Suite 120
White River Junction, VT 05001
(802) 295-6300
www.chelseagreen.com

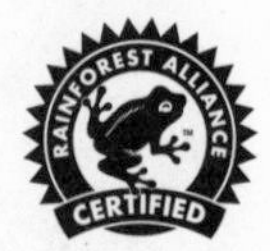

This book is dedicated to the mothers of chronically sick children.

Some would-be architects of our future look toward a time when it will be possible to alter the human germplasm by design. But we may easily be doing so now by inadvertence, for many chemicals, like radiation, bring about gene mutations. It is ironic to think that man might determine his own future by something so seemingly trivial as the choice of an insect spray.

Rachel Carson, author,
The Silent Spring, 1964

CONTENTS

Introduction ix

1. The Perfect Storm of Toxic Food, Sick Kids, and the Limits of Medicine 1
2. Going Beyond the Band-Aid to Help Chronically Sick Kids 11
3. Food-Focused Medicine for a Pharmaceutical-Heavy World 23
4. A Second Silent Spring (or, Good Intentions Gone Awry) 35
5. The Family Eating Modern Industrial Foods: Almost Everyone Is Sick 50
6. The Gut Microbiome, Symbiosis, and Dysbiosis 59
7. Unconventional Medicine for Treating Gut Dysfunction 74
8. Leaky Gut: A Key to Understanding Pesticide Impact on Health? 81
9. Chronic Exposure: Contamination as a Way of Life 93
10. The Making of Modern Industrialized Food 101
11. The GM-Food Debate: Controversy, Politics, and Truth 120
12. Going with Our Glyphosate-Filled Gut 137
13. Can Getting Rid of GM Foods Improve Mental Health? 157
14. Can Autism Spectrum Disorder Be Improved by Way of Gut Health? 169

15. Can Gut Health Improve Other Cognitive Problems? 178
16. Making Sense of Comorbidities in Children 183
17. Evidence-Based Medicine and Ecosystem Health: Why Not Ecomedicine? 191
18. Warrior Moms: The Call to Action 203

Acknowledgments 209
Resources 211
Notes 213
Index 245

Disclaimer

The information provided in this book is presented as helpful information on the subjects discussed. This book is not meant to be used, nor should it be used, to diagnose or treat any specific medical condition. For diagnosis or treatment of any medical problem, please consult your medical professionals. The publisher and authors are not responsible for medical conditions requiring professional supervision, nor are they liable for any damages or negative consequences from any specific health actions resulting from reading this book. References are provided for informational purposes and do not constitute universal endorsement of any website or other sources on the part of the authors or press. Readers should be aware that the websites listed in this book might change.

INTRODUCTION

In this book, we argue that a new generation of kids with chronic, hard-to-diagnose, hard-to-treat health problems is getting sick because of chronic exposure to poisons in the environment, and specifically in and from foods. Our children have guts that are impaired and immune systems that are overtaxed, making it hard for them to clear even the simplest health problems, such as colds. Eating processed foods that are high in carbohydrates, sugar, and hollow calories is the first problem, but in this book we argue it is not the *main* problem. The more insidious danger is foods that are full of pesticides, hormones, and antibiotics. How is it that at a time when we have the most efficient food production systems in the world, we are simultaneously putting ourselves at the greatest risk for food-induced health problems? In this book you will be offered one reason this is happening, what kinds of science can be relied on to make sense of it, and how food-focused medicine might be able to remedy these problems.

"What's making our children sick?" is a question we ask rhetorically, and without arrogance. In this book, we try to answer this question literally, and with humility. Children in the United States—and indeed, all over the world where a Western diet and industrial agriculture reign—are struggling with a new wave of chronic health problems that simply didn't exist several decades ago. We are not talking about broken bones and sprains, cuts and bruises, and coughs and colds that we *know* kids get all the time (some of which can be serious). What we are talking about in this book are chronic health issues that persist over years, problems that require long-term use of medical interventions and don't ever really go away. We are talking about problems that linger and are *managed* but have a huge impact on the quality of our kids' lives and the lives of their families.

What are these problems? Despite enormous strides in protecting the health of our children through medicine and public health,[1] today one in thirteen American children has a serious food allergy, a rate that increased by 50 percent over the last two decades.[2] Nearly 9 percent of our kids have asthma, with dramatic increases in rates from 1980 to today.[3] The prevalence of childhood eczema/atopic dermatitis in the United States is 10.7 percent overall and as high as 18.1 percent in individual states—again, a rate that nearly doubled in the past several decades.[4] More than 1.6 million Americans have Crohn's disease or colitis, and one in ten is a child.[5] One in roughly 140 Americans has celiac disease—a rate that has increased 4.5 times over the past fifty years, with rates increasing among children in particular, and this is before we get to gluten sensitivities.[6] Gastrointestinal reflux affects 8 percent of children, and today 10 percent of infants younger than twelve months with reflux now develop significant complications resulting in a disorder called gastroesophageal reflux disease, or GERD.[7] Irritable bowel syndrome (IBS) occurs in 6 to 24 percent of kids from middle school through high school.[8] Type 2 diabetes accounted for less than 3 percent of all cases of new-onset adolescent diabetes up until ten years ago, and now it accounts for 45 percent of these cases.[9] One in five American children is now obese. One in forty-one boys and one in sixty-eight children have a diagnosis of autism spectrum disorder,[10] 11 percent of our children have a diagnosis of attention-deficit/hyperactivity disorder (ADHD),[11] and just over 20 percent (or one in five) of our children either currently or at some point during their life will have a seriously debilitating mental disorder. These, too, are rates that have skyrocketed over the past two decades.[12] Finally, nearly 60 percent of our children experience chronic headaches, with 7 percent of these being chronic migraines.[13]

These numbers are staggering. What is happening to our children? Why are they so sick and with so many chronic, hard-to-treat ailments? Why have these problems shot up among children over the past several decades? What ties them all together? Looking at the numbers cumulatively, one might say that our children are experiencing an epidemic—an epidemic of complex, chronic ailments that doctors can do little about aside from minimizing the symptoms.

There are, in fact, no cures for many of these problems using the usual tools in the typical conventional medical toolkit. At best, doctors can treat the symptoms, eliminating the outward signs of disorder using strong medicines that suppress the body's reactions. But these often only work temporarily. Once the medicines wear off, the symptoms usually return. The underlying causes of these ailments are hard to eliminate partly because for many of these ailments we don't have adequate models of causation. Many of them have complex causal pathways that involve multiple physiological systems and sometimes multiple or cumulative triggers. As a result, parents of children with these disorders struggle to find help, not to mention even understand these conditions, and as a result bear an enormous weight.

Might it be that our children are in the midst of a health crisis that has yet to be named, yet to be fully understood? Perhaps we cannot name this crisis because we are looking at these health problems using old and insufficient models of disease and treatment. In fact, we argue it is possible that some, *if not all*, of these problems are related to similar underlying sources of pathogenesis (pathways to disease) that affect each child differently yet can be treated by way of some simple, low-tech, integrative medical interventions *starting with food*. In this book, we will provide the scientific and clinical evidence that supports this proposition.

We believe it is possible to look at health through a new lens that will enable us to tie these chronic health problems together and find a way forward. First, it is clear we need a vast transformation in how we live, and particularly in not just what we eat but how we provision ourselves with food—that is, we need to change what is in our food supply. Indeed, in this book we posit that the systemic health failures among our children are a result of something even more troubling than the physical symptoms in their bodies; they are the cumulative outcome of being born into and living in an environment that has been made toxic by agrochemical industrialized food production.

As a society that values and depends on the well-being of our future generations to thrive, we need to rethink the causes, complexities, and treatments for many of the chronic diseases on the rise today among our kids. Our children are sick because they are exposed to toxicants in the water, air, furniture, and petrochemical products they use. The amount of common household chemicals in use has been on the rise since World War II despite their known health hazards, and they are largely unregulated. But more than just toxic chemicals, our children are regularly exposed to toxicants that stress their developing immune systems, organs, and brains in even more insidious ways: through the so-called "healthy" food they eat. We will argue in this book that unless they are eating 100 percent organic food or homegrown vegetables from ecologically managed soil, they are eating toxic ingredients such as pesticides, hormones, and antibiotics. They are eating foods that are grown with, and contain, ingredients that are harmful to their health. One reason for this, among many, has been the rise in agrochemical technologies used to grow our food since the mid-1990s, including (though not limited to) use of genetically modified (GM), or genetically engineered (also called *transgenic*), crops that are designed to be used as, instead of, or in association with pesticides. We call this *industrial* food. *Modern* food is *industrial* food. GM technologies, although designed for the opposite outcome, have actually increased toxicants in our food environment. As a result of how we have "improved" our food production systems, our children today are now exposed to and end up consuming more toxic chemicals than any generation before them.

To be sure, this goes against the view of many conventional scientists, farmers, medical experts, and wide swaths of the public—those we call the *reluctant constituencies*—in relation to the effects of environmental toxicants (and particularly effects from GM foods) on our health. Their skepticism makes sense. Using genetic modification technologies with foods was, as mentioned, originally designed to *decrease* the need for toxic insecticides and herbicides (together called *pesticides*). In the wake of Rachel Carson's landmark book *Silent Spring*, great efforts were made to eliminate the deadliest of them: DDT. Even Rachel Carson was enthusiastic about the opportunities presented by genetic engineering to reduce toxic loads in agriculture. However, what we ended up with could not be further from her hopes.

In this book, we gather and present the evidence that the optimistic and necessary intervention to limit our use of pesticides has gone awry and, ironically, led to an *increase* in toxic exposure and pesticide use. This is having a huge negative impact on our health. In fact, GM food technologies are likely implicated, directly or indirectly, in the systemic biological problems that underlie many of the chronic ailments that we see in our children today. This includes crops that have been heavily sprayed with pesticides, and foods that have been turned into pesticides due to genetic modification. While a great deal has been written on the perils of industrial food production on the environment, as well as on the advantages of organic farming, few are connecting the dots between these insights and the health of our future generations.

Food-based chemical toxicants are finding their way into the blood and guts of our children, quite literally. We have a whole generation of kids who are growing up sick with chronic ailments and compromised capacities for living and learning. Survival for these kids means something totally different than it did for their parents and grandparents. The struggle for health (though never absent) now means dealing with allergies, asthma, rashes, digestive malfunction, and, in many cases, neurocognitive impairment. These, we believe, are related to chemical contamination that was meant to be harmless and is now vital to the industrialized production of our foods.

Industrial food production is just beginning to be understood from the perspective of the body's microbial ecosystem. We examine the evidence that chronic inflammation, aberrant immune responses, and, consequentially, chronic ailments are tied to persistent exposures to these chemicals. We are not alone in this position, though our perspective is far from mainstream. What we argue is that we are seeing in clinics across the country chronically afflicted children who suffer from being the unwitting participants in several decades of experimentation with agrochemically produced foods. This is an epidemic-scale health crisis.

Children carry toxic loads from the mattresses they sleep on, the soaps they use to wash their hands, their sunscreen, and their antibiotics. Add to that mix of toxic exposures the fact that much of their food is loaded with chemical toxicants, and you get very sick children—children who are being made sick from the inside out. And in order to get our kids healthy, we need to think of their problems in terms of a damaged ecosystem; healing them might actually require healing our environment and detoxifying our foods in order to detoxify their guts. We need an approach to health and healing that thinks about human survival in terms of environmental sustainability, a form of *eco*medicine, if you will, that places a focus on food.

What has been missing in mainstream conversations and critiques about industrialized food production is a map to connect the dots between the science and the symptoms, the data from animal studies, new knowledge about the microbiology of gut health, and the clinical experiences of doctors who are trying to stay one step ahead of these debilitating problems. Thankfully, there are leading-edge scientists and clinicians who, along with mothers and fathers of very sick children, are starting to make these connections. If you are one of those parents, or know parents like this, or if you are a physician trying to help these kids, our book is written for you.

The Collaboration That Produced This Book

Our approach to this problem is one that has grown out of collaboration between a clinician and an anthropologist. Dr. Michelle Perro is a food-focused pediatrician who has been practicing medicine for thirty-five years, the last fifteen of which have been in pursuit of integrative strategies that work to help kids with these troubling disorders. Watching the steady stream of ailing children, from infants to teenagers, who came to her clinics every day and realizing that her repertoire of remedies from medical school and her scientific journals was insufficient, Michelle began a journey into the world of integrative medicine focusing first and foremost on food. Poring over the literature and available evidence led her to a form of practice that was unconventional but was nevertheless rooted in biomedical knowledge and science. She turned to therapies that worked. This involved delving into the practice and art of functional medicine, homeopathics, and herbal medicine, and homing in on new scientific information from animal studies on food and health. All this led her to focus on what her patients were eating and drinking.

For Dr. Perro, this book distills the kernels of insight about our current predicament around food and health that have been gained over the past decades of research and sets them in conversation with her clinical experiences. *What's Making Our Children Sick?* explains how she deals with these problems head-on, and in ways that are not always (or not yet) established in clinical practice guidelines, with problems that begin (and sometimes end) in the gut.

Vincanne Adams is a medical anthropologist PhD who has spent much of her professional life exploring and comparing medical systems of Asia to those of the United States. Her journey into a critical exploration of the oversights and limits of Western models of health and healing began early on, as she witnessed efforts to translate Chinese and Tibetan medical therapeutics by biomedical science. Over the course of many years, she asked in various medical settings: What cultural, social, political, or economic insights have shaped knowledge, including scientific medical knowledge, and how do these affect health outcomes? She observed how certain forms of knowledge not only helped but also often obscured and obstructed health. Her study of Asian medicines also made her immediately familiar with and sympathetic to the notion that *food* could be both a cause of and treatment for disease, and she often wondered why it seemed so absent from Western medicine.

Although Dr. Adams was skeptical when she first heard about the possibility that GM foods and their associated pesticides were causing massive disorders in children, she recognized some of these health problems in children she knew. Hearing Dr. Perro talk about her typical patients, and finding in these stories an echo of patterns and pathways that could have been used to help many children, drew her into a commitment to learning more about Dr. Perro's work. Dr. Adams was intrigued—what exactly was integrative medicine and how were Dr. Perro's approaches to food different from those of other doctors she had met? The high rates of chronic health problems among kids might be correlated with the increase in use of GM technologies and their associated pesticides, but what evidence was there of a *causal* relationship?

After plunging deeply into the science of agrochemical food production, chronic health problems, digestive health, and the effects of toxic exposures—often reading over Dr. Perro's shoulders—Dr. Adams became more and more convinced of what Dr. Perro argued: Some foods were harming us and our children. More significantly, it became clear that what needed explaining was not only how food was implicated in poor health but also how science was being used (or not) in medicine, including the ways that politics influenced scientific knowledge.

In another line of her previous work, exploring recovery in post-Katrina New Orleans, Dr. Adams investigated the uneasy relationship of inequality between large corporations that controlled basic resources needed for human health and the most vulnerable members of the public who suffered from being denied access to these resources.[14] She began to see similar patterns of inequality in our agroindustrial food production systems, where large corporations held a monopoly not only on the products farmers needed for growing food but also on the science that was being produced to endorse use of these products. Avoiding conspiracy-theory logics, she plunged into the debates in the science and, together with Dr. Perro, they carved a path to the insights you will find here. Forming an alliance, they created a plan to write this book.

Tying together the connections between really sick kids and the politics of knowledge around GM food sciences first required learning more about Dr. Perro's patients. Over a two-year period, they interviewed patients and their families and created a set of case studies that they believed were representative of the larger epidemic. They then did more homework on the science, tracking down the old and new studies that provided evidence of these food-health connections. This also meant dealing with scientific data that were controversial and, in some cases, up for debate. They consulted with microbiologists, biochemists, geneticists, pediatric experts, and farmers to help make sense of these controversies. They attended workshops with organic food experts and interrogated the activists at the front lines of agroecology movements. Over time, these collaborative efforts produced enough material to write this book.

Not only do we see our book as a resource for others who are trying to connect the dots between agroindustrial food and poor health, but also we hope it offers a template for larger social and political change on issues of food health, children's well-being, and what we believe should be the future of medicine.

We have just begun to uncover some of the problem spaces in our current *zeitgeist*—a perfect storm, if you will—wherein some patients struggle to find cures for their very sick children and, in finding none, reach the limits of modern medicine. Patients and practitioners alike are forging paths into uncharted waters in the midst of this storm, creating integrative clinical practices that work, challenging the world of science, and engaging in politics for change. By turning to food-focused integrative medicine, people are finding answers and solutions. While conventional science moves at a snail's pace toward the kinds of tests and trials that we need to show the many causal links between GM pesticide-filled foods and chronic health problems, we believe we have no time to spare. Already there is plenty of good forward-thinking research that can help us start connecting the dots and filling in the blanks over our modern food predicament. Our children have been a living science experiment, and the evidence of its failure is our children's failing health.

We want to empower others who might or might not already be involved in the political effort to think about human bodies in the same way we must think about sustainable environments, in and through clean and nutritious food.

CHAPTER ONE

The Perfect Storm of Toxic Food, Sick Kids, and the Limits of Medicine

A mother of a critically ill child once said to me, "Children are easy—until they get sick."

JENNY PERKEL, author of "Parenting a Sick Child"[1]

Willa was a four-year-old when her mother, Sherrie, told us that her daughter had been sick "pretty much from the time she was born." Willa was a couple of weeks old and she had severe reflux.[2] So her doctor put her on Prevacid (at the time a prescription antacid designed to decrease acid in the stomach) at a few weeks old. Willa would breastfeed and then throw up everything, and she was in a lot of pain. Exhausted, her parents would try to lay her down . . . at which point she would vomit, and then scream. Start over. Repeat. "It was pretty awful, as I'm sure you can imagine," her mother said, "for a two- to three-week-old to be so miserable."

At that time, Willa's regular pediatrician recommended her mom take her to the large teaching hospital in the city. There, they did a barium swallow looking for blockages in her esophagus or anatomical anomalies, and a litany of food allergy tests. All of Willa's anatomy seemed to be fine, and her IgE tests (immunoglobulin E, produced when the body has an allergic reaction) showed nothing abnormal. And yet, there was no denying her pain and her struggle to keep food down. Over the months that followed, Sherrie painstakingly tried to nurse and, as the months went on, to mash her daughter's food so she could eat it, a process that continued for another year. She tried different foods, and continued with the Prevacid.

The Prevacid helped Willa a little bit, her mother told us, but not enough to make the symptoms go away entirely. And they couldn't get her off the medication. Every time they'd try to wean her off, she would go right back to not being able to keep anything down, and was still very uncomfortable. At the same time, she was having chronic ear infections. Every time she got a cold (and she got them often) she would get a really bad ear infection, which would then turn into a bad cough. Then she got bronchitis and pneumonia; in fact, Willa was on antibiotics for ten days almost every month. Eventually she was diagnosed with asthma.

By the time she was two, Willa had been on antibiotics *over twenty times*. Eventually Sherrie got a name for her daughter's problem: GERD, or gastroesophageal reflux disease. But she complained that all she got was a medicine for reducing Willa's symptoms. Neither the specialists nor her pediatrician offered an explanation or treatments that worked to get at what Sherrie called "the underlying problem."

Sherrie's voice was filled with a calm frustration cultivated over many years of struggle. Willa's chronic debilitating ailments were taking a toll. Summing up the obvious, Sherrie said: "Willa wasn't getting nourished. She couldn't keep down food. So, of course, her immune system wasn't strong, and she was susceptible to every flu, every cold that she was exposed to." Marking the visual evidence of Willa's decline was her growth chart. When she was born she was in the ninetieth percentile. She dropped completely off at seven months, and at nineteen months she was down around the third percentile. She was hardly growing at all.

When Sherrie finally came to see Dr. Perro, Willa was nineteen months old. When Dr. Perro saw her for the first time, she said to herself, "Wow, this kid is really sick." Dr. Perro was concerned that Willa was failing to thrive and not receiving the nutrients she required for normal growth and development. Although she was only two years old, taking her history was a lengthy process and included learning more about her parents' health. All of these factors informed Dr. Perro's treatment plan. The other striking thing about her case was the profound number of antibiotics she had taken in the course of her short life. This fact alone led Dr. Perro to think that alterations in her gut flora were a root cause of her symptoms.

Dr. Perro began the process of figuring out what was going wrong, starting with her gut. She did fecal testing because Willa was so little, rather than doing more blood work. She then started Willa on a program that would heal her gut and get her weaned off the Prevacid. Dr. Perro removed gluten from her diet because she knew that gluten was correlated with GERD in children. Dr. Perro also switched her to a completely organic diet, and gradually began treatment with various homeopathic remedies and probiotics based on how well Willa responded. It was a complex and multipronged process, but Sherrie went along with this approach.

The first results were immediate. Willa stopped getting the reflux. When dairy and soy were eliminated from her diet, her ear infections went away. "It was like a miracle," her mother said. Within a few more months, Willa started to grow. This was back in 2014. Since then, Willa continued to grow, and when we met her in 2016, she was normal height and weight for a child her age.

Public Frustration and the Turn to Integrative Doctors

The story of Sherrie's frustration in trying to help her daughter is one that is familiar to many. Families with children who have hard-to-diagnose, intractable, and often debilitating health problems are often thrust into a long battle, sinking resources of time, energy, and money to help them, frequently with very little to show for their efforts. Moms everywhere—and it is mostly moms—are telling us these stories. After a while, the stories start to sound familiar.

They are frustrated, exhausted, and angry. They can't get effective treatments. They feel let down by their doctors who, in fact, are often equally frustrated. Parents load their kids up with antibiotics only to learn that these are probably damaging their children's guts. One can imagine the confusion this produces. These moms feel helpless. And then they discover there are alternatives. When they finally meet a doctor who is willing to try something new, these moms are usually ready to try just about anything. Sometimes what they find out, often to their surprise, is that their kids' issues start, and many end, with the simplest medicine of all: food.

Sean, another patient whose mother we interviewed, had a similar story. He was a three-year-old with eczema over most of his body. He wasn't eating well. His mother, Irene, described the feeling she had when she realized that she hadn't had to buy Sean new clothes in over a year. "You know," she said, "on top of the eczema over nearly his whole body, I realized we did not need to buy clothes and I thought, that's not good. It's not good when your child is not growing." Sean was three but he was wearing clothes for an eighteen-month-old. Irene said, "You could put your fingers around his upper arm [she demonstrated by touching her thumb to her forefinger in a small circle]."

Irene had a hard time telling the story without getting emotional. "It was terrifying," she said, "to have a kid who was sick and to feel so helpless about it. I went to the pediatrician and I said, 'Oh my gosh, what do I do?'" and to her surprise, her regular pediatrician said, "Oh, that's not that bad eczema. We can put some steroids on it." Irene continued, "I mean, he was covered from head to toe in a rash and he says, 'That's not bad'!"

Irene described going to buy the "Costco-sized" tube of steroids for her son. She went home and started thinking about how skin is the body's largest organ and, even though her husband also had eczema, it seemed tragic to have to use the steroids on her three-year-old. She was infuriated that her physician had tried to minimize his symptoms by saying "That's not bad eczema. He's fine. He's just fine." Instead, Irene said, "Something is not right here. I had another child before this and he didn't have these problems, and there's something wrong. He's off."

Irene talked about feeling helpless, feeling like her doctor was not taking her concerns seriously. What most surprised her, looking back, was that he never mentioned food. In contrast, she described her first visit with Dr. Perro as an experience that was "like finding someone who spoke my language." Dr. Perro listened to Irene. She asked her what *she* saw. This was not another doctor who said, "He's fine." Irene felt seen, and heard, and finally in the right place, especially when they, together, started to figure out some underlying causes.

Dr. Perro and Irene started testing Sean for food sensitivities. His test results showed he was immunologically reacting to many foods: eggs, almonds, gluten, and dairy. Looking back on it, Irene realized that she was feeding Sean so many of the wrong foods, and it was hurting him. She had been feeding him dairy, yogurt, and eggs and then was told to get him off dairy. But when she switched him to almond milk, his symptoms got worse, and she realized he was also allergic to almonds.

When Irene talked about Sean's food sensitivities, she called them "allergies." Sean's regular pediatrician wouldn't call them that, nor would Dr. Perro. In fact, his pediatrician tested Sean's antibodies, and said the results technically showed no food allergies. The tests he ordered were designed to find the kinds of allergies that can make kids go into anaphylactic shock (the kind that produce IgE responses). What Dr. Perro looked for were more subtle immune responses, the kind that are often called food sensitivities (an area of medicine that is controversial). Food sensitivities show up as IgG and IgA antibodies, suggesting an immune reaction that is not viewed as a *true* allergy in conventional medicine, but that still shows an activated immune system.

The confusing part for Irene was that Sean's problems *did* present like serious allergies, even though he didn't test positive for IgE antibodies. Dr. Perro felt that his sensitivities could be implicated in his eczema and his delayed growth. She reasoned that these immune responses were likely related to underlying inflammation in his gut. Skin is just an external manifestation of what's going on in the gut, she told Irene. When Irene finally bit the bullet and eliminated the four things Sean was sensitive to (eggs, almonds, gluten, and dairy) from his diet altogether, Sean started to eat again, eventually with a strong appetite, and his eczema started to clear. Over time, Dr. Perro added in homeopathics for gut healing and restorative nutrients such as magnesium and zinc to correct his deficiencies of these minerals. Irene was tearful when she described it. Sean's symptoms started disappearing until they were largely gone. He was 95 percent better: "*Improvement* is not a strong enough word here," she said. "I mean, this was a child who *would not eat*, and now he is a child who *wants to eat everything*."

Over time, as Sean's gut started to heal and subsequently to digest properly, his eczema cleared up. The added bonus for Irene was that because she herself began following the same diet as her son, her own asthma improved dramatically. She described previously needing to use inhalers regularly, even ending up at the hospital several times a year. She described keeping a note by her bedside for her husband, just in case she needed it in the middle of the night. It read: *Don't panic. I am having an asthma attack and need to go to the hospital now.* Since removing dairy from her diet, however, she hardly needed to use her inhaler anymore. She went from needing it multiple times a day to only about once a week.

Irene felt like her world had been turned upside down. How was it that none of her doctors had ever mentioned a dietary shift? Here, it seemed, was an obvious culprit: dairy. The proof for her was in the outcome. Over time, with multiple visits for Sean, treatments for Irene as well, and her own sleuthing on the internet, she put it all together: They were getting sick from the food they were eating. But why? Dr. Perro explained to Irene that the foods we eat today are not like the foods we ate twenty years ago. Foods today have all kinds of contaminants in them, and these contaminants are toxic to the body, specifically to our guts. This is why so many more kids are developing food allergies, not to mention a whole slew of chronic problems.

Irene described looking at food in a whole new way since Sean's dramatic improvement. She told us how she now completely avoids toxic ingredients in foods, and only eats organic. We asked her whether she had a theory about how food caused ailments. She said it was a combination of things: pesticides in the foods, genetic modifications of the foods, the antibiotics in the meats and dairy, and then all the other processed or synthetic ingredients in the packaged foods. She said she reads labels carefully now: "There is corn, soy, wheat, and even dairy in everything. You have to read the fine print."

The Perfect Storm

To some readers, the notion that we are eating foods that are making us sick seems somewhat far-fetched. After all, we live in a country that has the most proficient and prolific systems ever known for the production of foods. We have a broader variety in our food choices than any generation preceding us, and foods are "cleaner" (in the sense of being free from microbial pathogens) than ever in history. On top of that, most middle-aged adults are likely to say that they ate all these foods even before something called "organic" existed, and they are not *that* unhealthy.

Yet it is clear that our kids are getting more food allergies, food sensitivities, and chronic health problems related to diet than ever before, and certainly more than we middle-aged adults did as kids. (Adults are not that healthy either, if you look at population statistics.) According to 2013 data from the Center for Child and Adolescent Health Policy, over half of US children and teens live with a chronic condition.[3] Approximately 40 percent of American children now have an allergy. This is remarkable in a nation that spends more money on its health care and provides more drugs on a per capita basis to its population than any nation in the world.

Is it possible that we are doing something wrong? Is it possible that all of these chronic problems in our kids are related to something so basic as *food*? Is it possible that the ways we are treating these problems through our existing medical repertoire are missing the mark in some part or altogether? We believe our kids are sick with chronic ailments today because of the cataclysm of at least three things:

1. Living in a toxic environment from chemical exposures, rather than from microbial infections, making the foods we eat a source of disease
2. Outmoded models of clinical care and disease causation
3. A scientific community that is embattled when it comes to food-health science

These ingredients create an uncomfortable brew. This is a terrain of conflict that results in poor health, frustrated patients and families, and conflicted medical professionals. We have, in other words, created a perfect storm for ourselves and for our kids. This storm starts with what we eat (and what we feed to our kids). It also moves beyond this very quickly.

What we are faced with today is more than just a problem of eating too many sugars and fats, too many fake foods, or what Michael Pollan, in his book *In Defense of Food*, calls *edible foodlike substances*—the packaged foods filled with secret ingredients or artificial man-made fillers. To be sure, these food choices are unhealthy, and there is ample scientific consensus on this opinion. What we are interested in goes beyond these well-known unhealthy foods. The big issue here is that our kids are not just getting sick from eating fake foods, they're getting sick from eating *real* foods, foods that many of us would consider *healthy*. Why? Because many of our real foods have been overloaded with fertilizers, pesticides, hormones, and antibiotics, and have been redesigned with genetic alterations that often lead to increased loads of toxic pesticides.

Our concern is that many of our so-called "healthy" foods contain the same toxicants that are found in fake foods. That is, many of the fruits, vegetables, and grains that we eat (or that our farmed dairy and livestock eat) have been chemically altered and industrially grown with the use of pesticides. These foods contain chemical toxicants either because of the ways they were modified or grown, or because of the fact that they were fed modified foods that we, in turn, eat. Modern food is now industrialized food that comes from a whole interconnected chain of agroindustrial chemical dependencies that pervade the entire food ecosystem. To sum up, we are concerned, specifically, with anything that is not *organic*. Organic foods are, by definition, foods that have attempted to avoid (usually successfully) these chemical production dependencies. (It is important to note that some organic foods can also be tainted and some are large-scale cash crops, but they remain the better choice and a good place to start.)

The Toxic Lunchbox and Beyond

What is happening to our kids today reaches far beyond the problem of food, even if it starts there. We are feeding our children toxicants, often without knowing it. Their lunchboxes are too often filled with foods-plus, foods that have added qualities that are harmful to our children's guts and, consequently, their bodies and brains. Widening the lens from the toxic lunchbox, we know that their ailments are symptomatic of our larger failure to understand the ecosystem within which our foods are grown and upon which we depend for survival.

Widening the lens even further, we know that harmful chemicals permeate not only the foods, but also the environments within which our children live, from the plastics in their cosmetics and school supplies to the particulate pollution in the air from cars and factories. All of these, cumulatively, are causing massive disruptions of our kids' health, an irony considering that the chemical revolution was once promoted as "a medical miracle" but is in reality a children's health disaster. This system is unsustainable. Our sick kids are the *prima facie* evidence for this.

If we begin our journey with the simple premise that many of our foods are making our children sick, we must quickly move to more deep-seated and hard-to-answer questions. First, how and why have our foods been turned into toxicants? Can these transformations in our foods explain all of these varied chronic disorders? What evidence can we rely on to make sense of the links here? What models of health and disease and, more importantly, of clinical practice are going to lead us out of the storm?

In this book, we address these questions systematically. In the chapters following, we intersperse clinical case studies with an exploration of the sad realities of industrial food production technologies that are likely linked to increased toxicants in our foods. We explore how recent biomedical sciences are laying the groundwork for food-focused theories of disease, focusing on the microbiome and leaky gut. We return to clinical cases before turning, in chapter 10, to the controversial debates surrounding genetic modification of foods.

When we return in the second half of the book to clinical cases, armed with our knowledge of a new medical model, we look at how organic food choices can improve not just digestive health but also neurocognitive health in a series of chapters about kids who have mental health issues. In chapter 11, we talk about what kind of medicine *food-focused medicine* is, and how it might address this new epidemic of chronic childhood diseases. We ask: Can we imagine a medicine in which the limiting factor for health is a healthy food environment? Might this medicine help us think in new ways about our food ecosystems as interdependent and mutually benefitting symbiotic species and systems? Is clean food an ideal mediator between the species that are needed for healthy environments and those needed for a healthy body?

We end our book with a tribute to the mothers who have engaged in the battle, alongside their clinicians, to tirelessly help their kids achieve health in a world that seems filled with obstacles to prevent this. We applaud their willingness to stay in the game, even when it means alienating themselves from family and friends and, sometimes, even jumping into the political battlefield to change the regulatory environment. Their tenacity is why we dedicate the book to these moms.

Let's start, then, with a look at some more clinical cases and the story of how Dr. Perro found herself needing to explore food as medicine.

CHAPTER TWO

Going Beyond the Band-Aid to Help Chronically Sick Kids

Tell me what you eat, and I shall tell you what you are.
JEAN ANTHELME BRILLAT-SAVARIN,
author of *The Physiology of Taste* (1825)

Trevor was a nine-year-old who had been diagnosed with ulcerative colitis. Like Willa and Sean, Trevor's problems also began early in life, when he was just a newborn. He contracted *E. coli* from a hospital procedure, and on his postcircumcision checkup, an attending physician noticed an adhesion and, without hesitating, ripped it open with his fingers. He then put the old bandage back on the wound.

His mother, Georgia, told the story with the precision of someone who had been traumatized—as if she had daily relived those moments of nearly nine years ago like a war veteran recalling a battle—there was blood everywhere. A few days later, Georgia said, Trevor developed encephalitis (inflammation of the brain). He was only one week old. The hospital put him on IV antibiotics and kept him in the hospital for three weeks, and when the physical symptoms subsided, they thought it was cleared. They sent him home, but in one week, the encephalitis came back. Trevor went on antibiotics again, this time for four weeks. So, for the first two months of his life, IV antibiotics and mother's milk were all he got.

Witnessing two bouts of encephalitis so close together, the pediatrician thought Trevor had an immune deficiency, which was not an unreasonable assessment. Georgia told us the story carefully, to make sure we understood her sense of injustice: The doctors thought there was something wrong with *him*, she said, rather than assuming it was just the same bug—the *E. coli* infection that *the hospital had caused* that had not fully cleared. Basically, they didn't want to admit they had discharged him too early. Their solution was to put him on IV immunoglobulin treatments once a month for a full year. Georgia described trudging once a month to the hospital for the IV treatments, sitting there with her poor son for hours. Trevor's health was already compromised; his eating and digestion problems started way back then, when he was just a newborn.

A few years later, scar tissue from the encephalitis in one of the ventricles of his brain was causing a blockage. He developed hydrocephaly —fluid was accumulating in the brain cavity, swelling and putting pressure on his brain as the fluid expanded between the tissue and his skull. He had to have emergency brain surgery to put in a shunt and drain the fluid. That procedure had to be repeated two more times as he grew, each time with major hospital stays.

Looking back, and relying on her avid commitment to searching the scientific literature that could explain her son's troubles, Georgia was now pretty sure that one of the reasons Trevor developed colitis when he was nine years old was because of these early and ongoing interventions. First off, she reasoned, there were the antibiotics in his first weeks of life, and then there were the repeat brain surgery procedures that not only involved more serious antibiotics but also other immune suppressants. His gut just never developed, she said.

Before we met him, Trevor had been on a course of prednisone (a steroid) and Asacol (an anti-inflammatory) for the colitis for several years. Still, his mom said, it just wasn't getting much better. The colitis would come and go; he'd have a few good weeks and then the chronic symptoms would come back. He'd have to get up three or four times a night to go to the bathroom, and when it was really bad, he'd stay home from school rather than suffer the embarrassment of having to make repeat visits to the bathroom all day long. "That's a lot for a little kid to handle," Georgia said.

Eventually, blood started to appear in Trevor's stool, so Georgia went back to the specialist. That doctor told her they should move up to *stronger* steroids. Georgia described being distraught over this news—she couldn't figure out why things were getting worse instead of better. She had arguments with the pediatrician and nurse practitioners, who were pressuring her aggressively to use the stronger meds. But, she said, she wanted to figure out what was causing the colitis in the first place, not just treat the symptoms. She described feeling like a wall was being thrown up between her and her son's doctors. When a friend recommended Dr. Perro, she said it was like finding a light at the end of the tunnel. Dr. Perro saw Trevor's problem from a totally different perspective. She got Trevor to start working with a nutritionist, gave him homeopathic remedies, and started to figure out his food issues. Dr. Perro's approach was clear: First, she aimed to figure out what factors triggered his colitis. She started in the gut, which, in Trevor's case, was the obvious place.

Under Dr. Perro's care, Trevor started on a series of treatments that would heal his gut. They took him off gluten, dairy, soy, corn, and sugar. Then, Georgia's father, who had done some sleuthing on the internet, told her that Asacol could have some of the side effects Trevor was experiencing, including aggravating the ulcerative colitis. At that moment, Georgia said, she realized that she was not sure she could trust Trevor's doctors at all, or that she would have to be willing to challenge their recommendations. She checked in with Dr. Perro about taking Trevor off the Asacol and about possibly switching to a different physician who was less confrontational than the one she'd been dealing with at the pediatric office. Still, both doctors agreed that Trevor could stop using the Asacol. The minute he did, nearly *all* of Trevor's symptoms subsided dramatically.

It was clear that the combination of changing his diet and getting him off drugs that seemed to be working against him was helping. What surprised Georgia the most was that during all of the time before she came to Dr. Perro, during her conversations with so many specialists, *not one* doctor suggested that any of Trevor's problems could be related to food. In fact, when she mentioned early on the idea of changing his diet, they told her a severe change in diet would *not* be good. The only thing his original doctors ever recommended was white breads and bland foods.

To Georgia, this seemed like the opposite of good advice. Most of those foods were high in gluten and sugar, which she knew caused inflammation. She told us all his doctors could talk about were the drug classes, starting him on the least potent and explaining that if things did not work with those, they would move to more potent drugs. Everything was about drugs, she said.

Instead of giving him more drugs, Georgia got Trevor off all the foods he couldn't handle. She also began to feed him an exclusively organic menu. Trevor's gut seemed to be getting better (although it was not an overnight success). Dr. Perro kept Trevor on the prednisone for a while, and with the changes in diet and homeopathic remedies, he got better and better. But he still couldn't shake the colitis entirely. It was 85 percent better—he only had to use the bathroom once a night, and he stopped having the long, severe episodes that kept him out of school. That alone was like a miracle. But the colitis would flare up on occasion. It was as if he just couldn't get over that last hump and get into remission.

Georgia told us that Dr. Perro figured they were not quite to the bottom of Trevor's issues. She described how instead of going back into more discussions of his gut, Dr. Perro started to look at the larger picture. She said that Dr. Perro seemed to *get* Trevor, that she could see him as a whole person, in his entirety. "This doctor," Georgia said, "she got that Trevor was a really worried kid—a kid who overworried. That was part of his problem." Georgia explained how the gut and brain were connected; gut problems could make Trevor nervous, but being nervous added to his gut problems.

Dr. Perro recommended Trevor see an acupuncturist and a therapist. The acupuncturist was great, Georgia said, and Trevor liked that treatment, but the therapist wasn't a good fit. Trevor wasn't comfortable talking about his worries, so Dr. Perro recommended an osteopath (a type of doctor who emphasizes body manipulation alongside other therapies). That helped more. Over the course of four months, Dr. Perro kept Trevor on a diet that had no gluten, dairy, corn, soy, or sugar and was only organic. Georgia then worked with all of her physicians to gradually wean Trevor off the prednisone. They gave him one last big push with the steroid and then began to wean him off. It all seemed to work, she said.

At the time Georgia was telling us her story, Trevor was off the prednisone and he had been symptom-free, in remission, for four months. "It would be hard to figure out which piece was ultimately responsible for the improvement," Georgia said. "In the end, I think it was all of them." Figuring out the food issues, getting him off the things he was sensitive to and onto the organics, but also getting him off the Asacol, onto the homeopathics, and the bodywork. It all worked together, in her mind, like a team.

Georgia's firm belief that Trevor's recovery lay largely in the healing of his gut pulled her toward this speculation: Could it be that he never developed a healthy microbiome early in life because of all the antibiotics? Could it be that his condition persisted because the drugs he was taking were not correcting that problem or perhaps making it worse by masking the real culprits? Could his inflamed and ulcerated colon have been not a cause but a *symptom* of a more fundamental pathology—such as being unable to digest the foods he was eating because his gut was compromised from the toxicants he was eating, including those in his foods and in his antibiotics?

Georgia kept returning to the fact that, through the whole thing, half the battle for her was finding the right kind of doctor. When she told the first pediatric gastrointestinal specialist about her work with both a nutritionist and Dr. Perro, including her use of homeopathics, she got a little pushback. "They basically disregarded all that," she said. They acted as if it was more of a useless nuisance than a serious approach to his problems. And then, she said again, they warned her *against* changing his diet. This was the most stunning bit of the whole experience, she noted. That they didn't acknowledge there could be a link between what he was eating, his gut, and the inflamed condition of his colon.

Still, Georgia was not hostile or angry. "You know they saved his life twice," she said, referring to the specialist doctors who had helped Trevor in the hospital. The drugs for her were double-edged, both the antibiotics and the steroids. They had saved his life but were also implicated in causing his problems.

Let Food Be Thy Medicine

Georgia's story of disappointment and frustration with her caregivers, along with her admiration for their interventions that saved her son's life on several occasions, reflects a common set of assumptions held by parents of children with chronic and hard-to-diagnose or hard-to-treat conditions. Conventional approaches can get them only so far, help them only so much, and then they hit the limits of what's conventionally possible, and that's where things fall apart (or where they finally come together, again depending on how you see it). Georgia's insights that the medicines and treatments had both saved Trevor's life *and* caused his problems are familiar to many families. Others share the sentiments of Sean's mother, Irene (from chapter 1), who started to lose faith in her physicians after they told her that her son wasn't *really* sick. Irene actually felt as if there was little to no point in taking Sean to her old pediatrician for anything anymore. It felt to her as if his pediatrician was not getting to the bottom of things; his pediatrician was just putting the Band-Aid on him and sending her home.

Parents' commitments to trying integrative medicine are frequently tied up in the complex misalignment between patient and practitioner in and around treatments. Irene's first pediatrician *did* have an answer for her: Use steroids. But it was not the answer Irene wanted. She wanted to know *why* her kid was sick, not what she could do to mask the symptoms, only to have them come back the minute they stopped using the medicine. Sherrie had a similar experience with Willa. As long as Willa stayed on the medicines, her symptoms were (sort of) kept in check, though not entirely eliminated, but the minute she went off the medicines, her symptoms came back in full force. In Sherrie's view it was as if the doctors were fine with reaching a "steady state" in which persistent use of medicines was the only option. Trevor's mother had a similar experience, perhaps made more dramatic by the severity and intensity of Trevor's ailments.

For these mothers, the turn to Dr. Perro came from a sense of having reached the limits of medicine itself, of having reached the limits of using pharmaceutical remedies that only masked, or suppressed but did not eliminate the causes of, these symptoms. Dr. Perro recognized her patients' disenchantment with their primary care pediatricians, although that was never her goal. Dr. Perro's preference was to return these kids to their primary care doctors after the kids got better. But this wasn't always possible. Once they started with Dr. Perro, they wanted to stay with her for the long haul. This is part of the problem, part of the perfect storm.

Hippocrates, known by many as the father and founder of modern medicine, said, "Let food be thy medicine, and medicine be thy food." We have traveled far from his insight today, as pharmaceuticals become more and more a replacement for food and food is seldom seen as a source of medicine in its own right. In fact, one might argue that the second part of his aphorism is all we do now; we let medicine be a replacement for food. Still, in all the cases we've discussed so far, food has itself been a part of the therapeutic regimen; food *is* a medicine. We need to return to this wisdom. But we also need to make sure that the food we eat is not dangerous or harmful to our health. The problem today is that few doctors are trained to think of food as a first-line remedy, and even fewer are made aware of the fact that many foods have become dangerous.

In fact, among the growing ranks of clinicians who become focused on food's enormous role in health, many do so because they have personal experiences that are similar to those of their patients or they have patients who present with things they cannot cure and so they go on a hunt for solutions beyond the guidelines they currently follow. Dr. Perro, for instance, started to look at food in relation to health because of patterns she was seeing in her clinic, coupled with her own son's ailments. Her attempt to sort out his problems led to her finding alternative approaches to his treatment. At the same time, she was exposed to some of the science that linked exposure to pesticides to many chronic ailments. Things all came together for her then.

Good clinicians everywhere do or want to do much of what Dr. Perro does. What separates her from some other physicians is her willingness to think beyond the conventional repertoire she was taught in medical school. She uses tests that are often only being used in science laboratories and in integrative clinics. She also uses homeopathy, a several-hundred-year-old medical specialty founded by German pharmacist Samuel Hahnemann.[1] Based on the principle that "like cures like," homeopathy offers a wide pharmacopeia of "low toxicity" remedies that are administered in very low doses to stimulate the body's ability to heal itself. Few doctors believe that homeopathy has any proven efficacy, and even those who will say they have seen it work are at a loss to explain why. Dr. Perro looks beyond diagnoses that fragment the body's ailments into discrete diseases and tries to look at the overall pattern, starting with the most basic of triggers for health and disease.

More than anything else, what makes Dr. Perro appear somewhat radical as a clinician is her willingness to focus so much on food, and on the possibility that even some of the so-called healthy foods our kids are eating are making them sick in a variety of different ways. Her belief in the benefits of organic, and the dangers of nonorganic, foods might be shared among many physicians, but few would emphasize it as a treatment program. This makes her unusual in mainstream, but not integrative, medicine.

The chips are stacked against the kind of medicine Dr. Perro practices. Food-focused medicine has never been mainstream, despite the fact that medical schools do not entirely ignore food, at least in the sense of nutrition. But there are larger reasons for the resistance to making food a centerpiece for clinical treatments. The oversized presence of pharmaceutical and biotechnological solutions has long crowded out the more simple (and affordable) promise of food in diagnosis and treatment. Even if doctors want to pursue these pathways, there are obstacles that come from health policy, health insurance plans, evidence-based medicine, and the temporal demands of health care delivery, all of which impact the logistics of clinical practice. We also know that food solutions require behavior modification in patients, and this is often a paralyzing challenge for clinicians. All of these things make it harder for doctors to think outside the box, as we will see in the next chapter.

Still, we think the time is right for turning our attention to food. In the effort to go beyond the Band-Aid to get to the root cause of our kids' chronic health problems, we think it is imperative that we reexamine our present food supply and its links to chronic illness. Recognizing this connection is, in part, what food-focused medicine accomplishes.

Dr. Perro's Story

After working for fifteen years in pediatric emergency medicine, I came to the conclusion that most of what we were taught in medical school was "Pill for Ill" medicine. I watched patients come and go with emergencies such as acute infections, complications from cancer, asthma attacks, breaks, lacerations, and autoimmune conditions. I began seeing a pattern of what I call "acute on chronic" disease.

What that means is, for example, I would see a kid in my clinic and I would diagnose him with an ear infection, a common problem in pediatric care. I would take the history on an eight-month-old baby and the mom would say something like, "Oh yeah, this is his sixth ear infection." Or, I would see a kid with pneumonia and hear, "Oh yeah, he also has chronic asthma and eczema." I would see endless numbers of kids with issues . . . and then I would learn that, "Oh yeah, he has some sort of neurocognitive defect"—sensory integration issues, auditory-processing issues, visual-processing issues, autism spectrum disorder. These diseases did not exist at the rates we are now seeing them twenty years ago.

I thought to myself: "What am I doing? I'm just putting Band-Aids on issues." I love acute care. But we have a medical system that is devised to evaluate and treat acute care, not this chronic stuff. So from that point on, I identified the two issues: that our health care system was not designed to manage chronic issues, and that we were not addressing the root issues causing the problems. And then I began my work in integrative medicine. I wasn't the only one seeing these patterns. Whole communities of clinicians were talking about this and trying to come up with solutions.

At about the same time this was happening, I was also raising my own children. The first thing that happened was my son got really sick. He had recurring health issues, including frequent upper respiratory infections, such as severe croup. A dentist figured out my son had gastroesophageal reflux from an oral exam, which I figured out was likely triggering croup. I took him to the pulmonologist and gastroenterologist at a prestigious children's hospital, and they had very little to offer him. At that time, I was working at a clinic where I serendipitously crossed paths with a physician who was also a homeopath. So, I took my son to see this physician and ended up trying homeopathics.

During a particularly frightening night when was my son was having trouble breathing, I gave him the homeopathic remedies that were recommended. To my surprise the remedies worked. When I realized that I gave my kid what I previously thought were just little sugar pills, and it cured his life-threatening croup in like . . . five minutes, I was taken aback. Croup is common. I had dealt with croup every single night of my professional career. So right away, I said, "What am I doing?" How could what looked to me like a sugar pill be medically helpful?

I realized then that there was a whole other system of health care out there that I had never heard about. I was from New York—skepticism was in my blood. But I was interested enough to learn more. I started studying homeopathy and eventually became qualified as a homeopath. Homeopathy became one more tool in my medical toolbox, along with all the other tools I had from my medical training.

At about the same time that this was happening, I was living in a town where there was a group of activists and concerned moms. In 2006, I was asked to help as an advisor in the environmental movement, mostly related to stopping the aerial spraying of certain pesticides in the county and in the state. These moms wanted a pediatrician aboard to get some scientific information for their platform that showed the health effects of spraying. I was reluctant at first. I didn't know much about it. So I started to go to the science; I had to learn more about pesticides. And through that work I was introduced to the concept of genetically modified food and the impact of GM foods and their associated pesticides on health. I realized that the research done on animals (which was sparse) was pointing to problems that were similar to those that I was seeing in children. For example, early research showed that GM feed affected rats' guts and immune systems in particular. I was witnessing similar patterns in children. (Experienced clinicians look for patterns!) But there was no scientific information or research available on how the genetically modified food and pesticides might be impacting children. I was horrified.

The great advantage I have is that because I am trained in conventional medicine, I can run all the diagnostic tests that a regular doctor would and more. I almost always run a series of one or more tests: blood tests, stool tests, food sensitivity tests, genetic tests, and tests for specific infections. I can get a good picture of what a patient's gut microbiome looks like. For some kids, I look at nutrient levels and environmental toxicant panels. I check for the presence of Lyme disease and coinfections. Often I am limited in how many tests I can run because the family cannot afford them and insurance will not cover the cost. I spend a great deal of time interviewing the mothers or caregivers about the medical and health history of their children and their families, about what sorts of dietary changes, diagnostic procedures, and treatments they can handle. I find out where they live and what kind of toxicants they might be exposed to. I listen carefully to what the mothers say about the symptoms, the patterns—the ebbs and flows—of each. I have mothers keep food diaries and symptom diaries. I go over their findings during office visits. I read and respond to their emails daily.

CHAPTER THREE

Food-Focused Medicine for a Pharmaceutical-Heavy World

Twenty years ago, I think we knew about 10 percent of what we need to know about nutrition. And now we know about 40–50 percent.

DARIUSH MOZAFFARIAN,
dean of the Tufts Friedman School
of Nutrition Science and Policy[1]

In chapter 1, we talked about the perfect storm in medicine today—the cataclysm of (1) living in a toxic environment that makes the foods we eat a source of disease, (2) outmoded models of clinical care and causation, and (3) a scientific community that is embattled when it comes to food-health science. The perfect storm we are describing has as much to do with the notion that we are living at a time of environmental crisis as it does with *the clash of clinical and scientific cultures* that so many mothers with sick kids confront.

Currently, there is a huge gap between public supporters of medical theories about food health and the medical experts who largely remain rather skeptical about the scientific evidence in this area. The gap is caused by conflicting scientific claims. It is also, as we have said, caused by the fact that conventional doctors are not taught much about the pitfalls of our food supply. They are taught a great deal about pharmaceutical solutions to health problems, or what Dr. Perro refers to as "Pill for Ill" medicine. Pharmaceutically driven medicine tends to diagnose by way of the drugs that are available for treatment. Don't get us wrong, we know that miracles have been created by biotechnology and pharmaceutical research. From antibiotics to the wide repertoire of chemotherapies targeting specific forms of cancer, we have much to be grateful for when it comes to the pharmaceutical sciences. We also know that a great deal of medicine is not driven by pharmaceutical practices but by advanced technologies of diagnostics and therapeutics (think of surgeries and transplants). At the same time, however, a large portion of our treatments for chronic problems are pharmaceutical, and the hermetically sealed loop between "having a drug to treat symptoms" and "diagnosing for the drug" seems impenetrable. But pharmaceutical therapies targeting chronic, and sometimes debilitating, disorders don't do much more than mask symptoms. Yet we keep assuming that for these disorders pharmaceutical solutions will be sufficient.

Consider, for example, how many advertisements on television are for chronic digestive disorders (from IBS to constipation). Why would we continue to assume that pharmaceutical remedies are our only recourse for therapy when the most powerful contributor to our digestive health is on the table in front of us, in the foods we eat? One answer is that the pharmaceutical industry currently drives the funding for scientific studies in medicine, and this industry cannot (or doesn't usually want to) fund what it cannot benefit from financially.

Food-focused doctors are right there in the middle of this battle, often making the argument that we need to think outside the constraints of pharmaceutical medicine and to scour the scientific literature to see what might be helpful for patients with chronic disorders, alongside or sometimes in lieu of typical pharmaceutical approaches. In fact, it might be that intestinal dysfunction is the underlying source of other chronic health issues seen in kids, from autoimmunity to mental health problems. It might make sense, then, to always consider gut health in any diagnosis, but especially in chronic conditions, and this, in turn, should lead to a focus on food. But we are getting ahead of ourselves. Let's first explore what we mean by food-focused medicine and situate it in the context of integrative approaches more widely. Then we can turn to the links between toxic food and chronic illness.

It is important to remember that the embrace of integrative approaches to health, and particularly to food-related health, is not new. Food-focused medicine forms a small subset of the enormous field of practitioners who make up the world of conventional and unconventional approaches in medicine. For one reason or another, however, food is not usually seen as a primary source of pathogenesis or of treatment in mainstream medicine today for anything except a small sliver of diseases (although these diseases are widespread, including celiac, obesity, diabetes, cardiovascular disease, food intolerances, and allergies). The use of pharmaceuticals rather than food for therapy might be because of the way modern medicine has evolved in our country in close collaboration with the drug industry.

The notion of what constitutes "a nutritious diet" as it has been taught in medical schools over the past decades has been widely debated. Some guidelines, graphically depicted as "food pyramids," were introduced in the 1960s in response to rising rates of cardiovascular disease. Those pyramids have been revised multiple times since then and have also come under more scrutiny as questions about the role of the food industries in creating the guidelines has been brought to light. Also, advertising shapes our popular understanding of nutrition. This might or might not be beneficial. For instance, the advertising campaign to convince the American public that breakfast is the most important meal of the day was sponsored by Quaker Oats.[2]

Much of our knowledge of what constitutes "healthy food" and a "healthy diet" is changing today. New research on the role of the microbiome in health is forcing us to rethink the role of gut health in relation to overall health, even mental health. And, naturally, efforts to explore gut health are refocusing attention on the role of food in creating and sustaining a healthy microbiome (as we will discuss in chapter 6). But shifting the model is not happening fast enough. There is something of a lag in the transfer of useful information from the halls of science into medical schools or American Medical Association clinical guidelines, but even beyond that, the research is simply not there yet to start an overhaul of curricula or clinical guidelines in most medical schools. This, in turn, has a lot to do with the fact that we call our medicine "scientific." That fact also has an interesting history in relation to food.

A Cursory History of Scientific Medicine

The history of scientific medicine is variously told as one of either of these stories: (1) Medicine is becoming more and more rigorous and more effective through scientific and political regulatory processes, or (2) medicine is becoming more and more controlled by biomedical industries and pharmaceutical, market-driven concerns that have pushed far beyond health. Both of these histories are true; however, both versions of the rise of scientific medicine marginalize food-focused medicine in comparison with drug-driven medicine.

For instance, in 1910 the Carnegie Foundation commissioned a study of medical schools at a time when a wide variety of clinical practices were available, including osteopathy, electrotherapy, naturopathy, and homeopathy. This resulted in what was called the Flexner Report, which led to the scientific standardization and accreditation of medical school education, and criminalized alternative therapies, including homeopathy. It also consolidated the collaboration between pharmaceutical industries and the American Medical Association (AMA). The effort to regulate the sale of nonpharmaceutical products and more natural types of therapy (what the AMA called *potions and elixirs peddled by traveling medical men*) had been a concern of the AMA for decades. The Flexner Report thus led to wholesale marginalizing of therapies not produced by pharmaceutical companies, including those that more closely resembled *foods* than *drugs* (such as cod liver oil or omega-3-rich oils from the snake, hence "snake oil").

By the 1960s and 1970s the Food and Drug Administration (FDA) and the AMA together, in response to concerns over consumer demands for nutritional remedies as a type of food faddism, launched the Campaign Against Nutritional Quackery and subsequently implemented drug- and food-labeling requirements.[3] The requirements that were established in the 1960s not only criminalized nonapproved therapies but also drove many of them underground or into the world of nontherapeutic retail sales as "nutritional or food supplements."

The twentieth century was a time of consolidation of pharmaceutical sciences in American medicine, as Paul Starr documents in his 1984

Pulitzer Prize–winning book on the topic, *The Social Transformation of American Medicine*. After the Flexner Report, the subsequent rise of the scientific medical research industry over the decades following drove pharmaceutical and technology innovation to the forefront. Post–World War II innovation in medicine, coupled with the prewar discovery of sulfa drugs (the first antibiotics), led to the idea of *magic bullet* medicine, in which pharmaceutical therapies were able to eradicate most medical problems with the speed, accuracy, and effectiveness of modern firepower. By midcentury, medicine had become a highly technical science orchestrated around the work of laboratory research, and pharmaceutical industries became the driving force behind not just medicine but also medical education and basic clinical guidelines. The basic ways that physicians were taught to both conceptualize the body and treat its ailments gradually became more and more drug-driven.[4] The tight relationship between pharmaceutical research and clinical medicine that began in this era has persisted into the new century with only small interruptions of critique or alternative thinking, especially when it comes to food.[5]

Georgia's description (in chapter 2) of the advice she got for her son Trevor's colitis is a good example of this. Rather than considering the food Trevor was eating, his gastroenterologist's approach was to consider which drugs could be used to suppress his symptoms. And when asked for advice about diet, Trevor's physicians recommended one that was clearly nutrient deficient. More extreme examples of how pharmaceutical culture shapes medical practice come from a wide range of diseases. Kids with chronic constipation are prescribed drugs made of propylene glycol, a petroleum-based laxative, which has potential side effects on the kidneys through its metabolites. There are useful food remedies that might work just as well, including increasing fibrous foods and vegetable intake and decreasing dairy intake. Another example is migraine headaches, which are often treated with sumatriptan, even though riboflavin (a B vitamin) might also work.

The epidemic of digestive disorders in the United States, from IBS, inflammatory bowel disease, and chronic diarrhea to heartburn and GERD, has created a gold mine for pharmaceutical companies, but there is seldom much consideration over the role of foods in these digestive problems. This is shocking, considering food is the single most prolific ingredient in the digestive tract at any given time. Add to this the possibility that foods might contain a potpourri of harmful chemical ingredients, and the problem is multiplied. Current clinical guidelines are simply not attuned enough to the role of foods in diagnosing and treating these problems.

Again, the enormous benefits that have come from the development of a huge arsenal of pharmaceutical products that work to keep people healthy should not be dismissed. We only have to consider our own family histories, the stories of our grandmothers who lost one or more children before the age of five, whose brothers and sisters might have died before the age of sixty from diseases we can now cure. At the same time, however, we have to account for the omissions and effacements that have also emerged with this huge emphasis on pharmaceutical forms of care, especially when it comes to chronic disorders. One of these is the problem of side effects. Another is the marginalization of food in the clinical repertoire. Finally, more often than not, for people with chronic diseases, pharmaceutical solutions remedy symptoms but don't eliminate the cause of the disorder. Without being too cynical, we feel it's important to note that keeping people on long-term medications is an obvious financial boon to pharmaceutical companies.[6]

One of the interruptions in this history of pharmaceutical domination occurred in 1993, when a Harvard clinician named David Eisenberg pointed out that the average American spent more out-of-pocket money on complementary and alternative healing modalities than on regular "scientific" clinical care.[7] The move to alternative forms of care was frequently prompted by pharmaceutical medicine failures. This huge out-of-pocket expenditure included the fact that most people had insurance to pay for their regular clinical care. Eisenberg's data created a watershed moment—a moment that shed light on the growing levels of frustration American patients had with their conventional treatment options. The public was voting with their collective pocketbook, by seeking treatments they believed worked even if they were not validated by conventional medicine. Of course, many of these options included use of products that were not part of the FDA-approved pharmaceutical repertoire, such as supplements, herbs, and homeopathics. Some of these approaches were focused on food, or at least on supplements that factored in nutrition as a key to health.

The medical community also began to ask questions. Was this shift to alternative and unconventional therapies a sign of collective gullibility? Or were these treatments and models of therapy actually useful? In response to these and other questions, the federal government invested large resources into more research on the efficacy of alternative and complementary therapies. In fact, through the 1990s, it created a new branch of the National Institutes of Health to explore them—eventually named the National Center for Complementary and Alternative Medicine, and later changed to the National Center for Complementary and Integrative Health.

Out of this ocean of interest and investment, including numerous clinical trials on specific therapies over several decades, emerged the field of *integrative medicine*. No longer were the so-called alternative therapies solely the province of alternative doctors who often received a great deal of skepticism from other physicians.[8] Integrative medicine aimed to create pathways for conventional doctors to *integrate into* their practices healing modalities, models of health, and treatment protocols that were at the margins (or sometimes entirely off the map) of conventional care. Early on, the use of probiotics was an example of this approach. Today, use of probiotics is mainstream.

In the contemporary moment, many major medical institutions in the United States have integrative health centers of one sort or another. Modalities ranging from acupuncture and Chinese herbals to reiki therapy and mindfulness meditation are used in these centers, and clinical studies attempting to prove their efficacy continue to be rolled out. There is a growing body of evidence to suggest that some, though not all, of these therapies work quite well, particularly in conjunction with conventional medicine. These efforts offer testimony that our medical institutions are adaptable, evidence-driven, and accountable to not only the public but also to the notion that clinical outcomes matter. Still, at most of these centers all over the United States, much is up for debate.

What is perhaps most surprising is how seldom the topic of food arises in the integrative models of health and healing, not to mention in the research, these centers promote. It is not *entirely* absent, but when food comes up it is usually because there is an integrative doctor who is trained in functional medicine in the room. Often this type of doctor is someone who studiously tries to avoid thinking solely in terms of simple substitution models with alternative treatment protocols (e.g., substituting acupuncture for painkillers, mindfulness stress reduction for antianxiety medications, or using what is sometimes called a *green pharmacy* approach). Usually this doctor is someone who is less interested in single modalities of therapy (and testing them for specific diseases or ailments) and more interested in advancing a holistic approach to health, often starting with food. The integrative approaches we are interested in offer new models of diagnosis and treatment that explore systems biology, or how the body's various systems work together, holistically, including focusing on how digestive systems matter in relation to overall health. In some cases these treatments work better than conventional treatments for chronic problems.

It seems strange that food-focused approaches to health and disease would be considered "integrative" or "alternative." Food should be a major focus for all medicine. But even as public health policies embrace the problem of nutritional-related diseases as epidemic, there is little research on food, *let alone on the contents or nutritional quality of modern industrial food.* As new research on the microbiome grows, however, this could change. That research is telling us that the human gut is perhaps one of the most important keys to health. In fact, some researchers are saying the microbiome itself should be considered a human organ. But even as research in this area is exploding (for example, in May 2016, the White House announced the National Microbiome Initiative),[9] there is still surprisingly little research on food in the sense of bridging the gap between those who are studying industrial food production techniques and their ability to supply our populations with healthy food. One would think research on the microbiome would automatically direct our attention to food-health relationships, but much more funding is available for the study of genetics and developmental biology in relation to the microbiome than is available for the study of the effects of modern food on health.

Research on the microbiome is, nevertheless, generating some important insights. We now know, for instance, that antibiotics can create an unhealthy gut microbiome and that dysbiosis (we'll hear more about this later) can result from an imbalance of healthy versus unhealthy gut bacteria. But we also know that no matter what medicines are doing in the gut (for better or worse), and no matter what the genetics of gut inheritance are, most of us also *eat* between two and three meals a day. What we feed ourselves holds the greatest capacity to nourish us or, as the case might be, to harm us. It seems obvious that we should be studying what impacts different foods have on gut health. What little research exists is only now emerging, and we have yet to see its impact on how we think about clinical medicine. Knowing this, it is not surprising to learn how little doctors are actually taught about food.

Why Aren't Food and Nutrition More Present in Medicine?

To be sure, not all doctors or even integrative doctors are taught about, or even care much about, food. It is not missing entirely, but typically, doctors learn the basics of food in the form of nutrition courses or specific lectures on food-related disorders in medical school. They are taught to understand how foods are broken down in the body into basic proteins, carbohydrates, minerals, and vitamins and how the body needs and uses these basic biochemical ingredients. They learn cursory information about disorders with obvious links to food, such as Type 2 diabetes, obesity, cardiovascular diseases, and life-threatening food allergies. For example, they are instructed on the relationship between a low-salt diet in patients with hypertension and about the importance of moderating sugar and carbohydrate intake in patients with diabetes. They are taught to tell their patients about the merits of a well-balanced and nutritious diet. They know that too much sugar, trans fat, and nutrient-deficient or empty calories can lead to morbidities. But they know little to nothing about how food, specifically modified food, can also produce massive malfunction in the body's biological systems.

Few physicians today are taught much about the fact that many of the foods available to us *are not real foods* (or not *entirely* real foods). Nor are they systematically taught much of anything about what foods that have been grown with toxic ingredients or with added antibiotics and hormones are doing to our kids' bellies and bodies. This is not surprising. It is invisible partly because that information is not widely available, and what is available is often considered controversial. It is also invisible because we have not considered food a problem for long enough. It takes years, if not decades, for good research to find its way into the guidelines for good clinical practices. It takes even longer if we are not funding research on these important things or if the industries that fund most research have little to gain financially from this kind of medicine. Finally, it is difficult and expensive to do food research on human subjects and hard to track the data and turn it into firm results, a problem we will revisit later.

For clinicians like Dr. Perro, there are practical implications to the lack of fuller clinical guidelines concerning food. For example, when working with Trevor, who had ulcerative colitis, she spent many visits with the family discussing and planning his diet. Her frustration would mount when Trevor would return from a visit with his pediatric gastroenterologist and tell her that he said Trevor could eat all the white bread he wants, or that diet had nothing to do with his disease. The family was made quickly aware that they were caught in the middle of a food battleground.

The battleground is not defined merely by the difference between types of practitioners. The battleground also is formed by conflicting information about food's relationship to health. Many clinicians are not so much *dismissive* as *realistic* about food concerns on grounds that beyond the known repertoire of food-related ailments, there is insufficient science on the contamination of foods with toxic chemicals. Much of the available research on food safety, for example, is performed by agrochemical companies that produce the food, rather than by regulatory agencies that are charged with protecting our food supplies. But even regulatory agencies that know about these matters seem to be convinced that at present we are not exceeding safe levels of toxicants in our foods. Thus, questions about the reliability of this research abound.

We also know that trying to get people to change their diets is one of the hardest types of therapies to implement in the medical arsenal. Doctors, unanimously, will tell people to lose weight, exercise more, and reduce stress. Sometimes this will include suggestions about diet. They know, though, that most people find it very hard to change bad habits, particularly around food. It is even hard for doctors to convince patients to change their food behaviors when the deleterious effects of those foods are staring them in the face, so to speak. So, if there is a pill doctors can give for the symptoms—to reduce the deleterious effects, to undo the damage of the food—and if that pill is backed by clinical evidence of its effectiveness in doing these things, clinicians will often offer that pill before counting on patients to change their diets. Patients themselves will often *ask* for the pill in order to avoid having to make behavioral changes that might seem hard to sustain.

But what if our biggest food culprits are not the obvious ones? What if it is not just the high–trans fat, high-sugar processed foods that are overconsumed and habitually entrapping people? What if the food culprits of today are also hidden ingredients in the other foods we eat: the meat, dairy, poultry, grains, fruits, and vegetables that are produced with excessive amounts of toxic chemicals? If it is hard to convince patients to change their obviously bad eating habits, imagine how hard it is to wrap our collective clinical interventions around what we assume are "good" eating habits.

Greater understanding of the relationships between foods and health begs for clinical attention and research in all these directions. Such research and clinical guidelines are needed because, as we've noted, food-related health problems are on the rise—from food allergies and food-induced diseases to the numerous disorders tied to unhealthy diets. Is the fact that our food is saturated with chemicals that our bodies cannot tolerate a reason for this rise? What we need are efforts to study how many chronic disorders are also likely associated with gut dysbiosis, missing microbes, and the not-fully-understood interactions among food, dysbiosis, and genetics. Are problems of intestinal permeability involved in inflammation and disorders of the immune system, and could these explain the rise in so many autoimmune disorders? These questions are what we call attention to in this book.

Clinicians who are paying attention to these things are out there. We call these doctors and nurses, nutritionists, and integrative practitioners *food-focused*, or *food-forward, clinicians.* This is the niche that Dr. Perro finds herself in.

What happens when patients hit dead ends with their conventional clinicians? What happens when they realize that the models of care they've been taught to adhere to are not only *not* helping but might, in fact, be hurting them and their families? What happens when the pills stop working or don't work at all? For many patients, these dead ends force them to change their food habits. But what happens when the doctors don't think the problems are related to food? What happens when these patients start to read internet sites that offer other solutions, food-oriented solutions, and their clinicians dismiss their concerns? How do these patients and their families reconcile themselves when clinical models collide? How do practitioners handle the conflict and the controversy? Again, this is where the perfect storm occurs.

We are interested in these cases. We are fascinated with the challenge presented to clinicians in cases like this. What can be done and where can clinicians go to get reliable information about the things their patients are talking about? We are swimming in a sea of information and yet we, just like other clinicians and patients, find ourselves with a scarcity of truth on these things. While the internet provides an oversupply of information (which, of course, includes misinformation), few clear answers about the connections between foods and these intractable chronic health problems are available in the peer-reviewed journals. This is yet another reason why so little information on these topics finds its way into the clinical practice guidelines that doctors must follow. Thus, we are compelled to explore what a food-focused, scientifically grounded medical response to these problems might look like. This is why we wrote this book. So, what is the evidence that some of our foods are toxic, contributing to an epidemic of chronic disorders in our children?

CHAPTER FOUR

A Second Silent Spring (or, Good Intentions Gone Awry)

How could we have ever believed that it was a good idea to grow our food with poisons?

JANE GOODALL, author of *Harvest for Hope: A Guide to Mindful Eating*[1]

It could seem radical to consider that our food might be killing us, but in reality, although food is probably *the most important gift* we can give to our bodies, it is also the most probable source of its ailments. Food is the major route by which the environment is able to enter the body and by which the body, in turn, is able to transform nature's elements into ingredients that it can and must use to live. For this reason alone, it behooves us to think collectively about how to keep the environment healthy, and also how creating a toxicant-filled environment will likely produce toxicant-filled bodies. Just how, then, have we given the environment the capacity to provision us with toxic rather than healthy foods?

When we talk about how foods are contributing to the rise in chronic, persistent, and hard-to-diagnose health problems in our children, we are not talking about the typical food pathogens such as *E. coli* or rotten foods, foods that contain infectious parasites that find their way into the gastrointestinal tract and cause mayhem. What we are talking about is foods that many of us assume are healthy. This includes foods that we buy in grocery stores that come in nice sealed packages that have a long shelf life yet testify to their cleanliness and purity, sometimes even by being labeled "natural" and "healthy." But it also includes our fresh foods that *don't* come processed and in boxed up, man-made containers—that is, meats, dairy, fruits, and vegetables. But let's step back first and look at the ones we already know are bad.

From canned goods filled with high-fructose corn syrup to packaged foods made from soy, corn, refined wheat, and various trans fats, there are numerous ways that foods packaged for long shelf life are not healthy, even when their labels or our cultural ideas about them say they are. Many nonfoods and unnecessary food additives are in these products that have become part of the typical American diet. Again, these are the *edible food-like substances*[2] that Michael Pollan warned us about. Sandra Steingraber, who wrote *Raising Elijah*, also reminds us that these foods are the logical end point of our industrialized food production system.[3] But we are not only talking about these, or even the more typical killers—the ones David Kessler warned us about that create high-sugar, trans fat forms of addiction, or that Gary Taubes warned us about that result in epidemics of clogged arteries and diabetes, among other things.[4] These are all putting us at risk for sure. But what if the ingredients we think of as *healthy* that are inside of the packaged foods (the natural ingredients like corn, wheat, and soy) are also dangerous? What if, further, the nonprocessed foods—the fruits and vegetables and meats and dairy products that we find on the outside rows of the supermarkets—are also unhealthy? Is it possible that even if we stick to the *real* foods on those aisles we might still be at risk?

In this book, we will argue that in addition to the known problems associated with processed foods, which have been well documented and are generally accepted by the medical community as unhealthy, a remaining underlying cause of poor health in our kids might be exposure to toxic substances in and through *real* foods. We are talking about fresh dairy and meats that often contain high levels of antibiotics and endocrine-disrupting hormones. We are also talking about fresh vegetables, grains, and fruits that now more than ever are likely to contain toxicants because they were saturated with pesticides as they were grown. Some of these vegetables, grains, and fruits have actually been turned into pesticides in their own right, and we are convinced they pose a risk. What if that extra serving of vegetables turns out to *not* be what's best for your kid, after all? How can this be? And, if not *real* food, then what can we eat?

What we are specifically interested in in this book are foods that are grown under conditions of industrialized food production—techniques that have been honed for the past century to prioritize profitability and quantity by way of chemical enhancement. These foods, which we are calling modern or industrial foods, are distinct from both the kinds of foods we produced before biotechnological innovations from the 1970s to the 1990s and the kinds of foods one can get from local, organic farmers today. Foods grown under conditions of conventional agrochemically dependent industrialized methods are, we argue, disruptive to the body in ways that are still being discovered. How did this happen?

The Rise of Chemical Toxicants in Our Food

We have come a long way since Rachel Carson's scathing indictment of the use of toxic pesticides like DDT in her book *Silent Spring*. She showed not only that DDT ended up killing many species of insects far beyond those targeted for crop security but also that the chemical entered into the food chain, ultimately ending up in the fatty tissues of animals and humans, where it caused cancer and genetic damage. In part because of her work and her modeling of ecosystem impacts, along with the work of many other activist scientists, the large-scale use of DDT was banned in the United States in 1970.[5] From that point onward, the public debate turned for the first time ever toward questions over *which* pesticides were dangerous and which were not. Simultaneously, responsibility for proving safety of pesticides shifted from public opponents engaged in political activism to the chemical manufacturers and agroindustry businesses themselves. As a reminder, when we say "pesticides" in this book, we are using the term in a categorical way; it includes insecticides, herbicides, and fungicides and other chemical means of killing or eliminating agents that put food crops at risk. Many of these chemicals used to grow conventional food (even before we get to synthetic fertilizers, an entirely different danger), along with the genetic modifications to the foods themselves, have a short history.

The watershed moment generated by *Silent Spring* in American agricultural history led, in ways that might seem ironic today, to advancements in technologies and chemicals that were used to ensure both safe crops and *safe ecosystems*. That is, as regulatory agencies were tasked with providing public assurance of the safety of pesticide technologies in response to public outcry over things like DDT, agrochemical industries tried to improve on their own track records. Agrochemical companies tried to eliminate the worst offenders and come up with tactics that were, in theory, less harmful.

One of the most significant tactics to help farmers avoid having to use the toxic chemicals (and to avoid widespread exposure more generally) was the use of a technology that was developed not too long after the banning of DDT: genetic engineering. Genetic engineering (also called genetic modification, GM or GE, to produce transgenic crops called GMOs) is a scientific modification of a crop to ensure it is resistant to fungal or animal enemies or resistant to weed killers. That's right: *Agribusiness companies originally invented GM technologies in part as a response to the ban on poisonous pesticides like DDT.*[6] To be sure, their motives were not entirely pure. The growth of plant biotechnology was also a response to earlier transformations in the chemical industry; notably, their recognition of the declining supply and rising cost of petrochemicals in the early 1970s, which forced these companies to explore new avenues for research and product development. Agribusiness was seen as an ideal new target of opportunity not only because of the potential need for chemical products but also because of the perception that, because of population growth, the world's food supply would soon be depleted.[7]

Turning their attention to biotechnology, these chemical companies gave birth to a new kind of agriculture that would be dependent on both *biological and chemical* sciences and resources. The biotechnology that was born in this era was seen by many as solving anticipated global food problems. In fact, some of the scientists working on these technologies considered themselves forward-thinking ecologists, such as Howard Schneiderman, the scientist from University of California (UC) Irvine and Washington University in St. Louis, who went to work for Monsanto in 1975, where he developed biotechnological approaches to genetic engineering. One of his early papers developed the notion of *planetary patriotism*, a model for saving the planet while also, patriotically, protecting our planet's food supply.[8]

Right off the bat, though, others saw these mergers as a risky extension of our dependency on chemical pollutants that were already showing signs of harm. While arguments were made by some that these new products and biotechnologies would reduce the need for harmful chemicals, other scientists who had long been entrenched in the battle against chemicals saw the birth of these biotechnologies as yet another guarantee of future dependency on a range of agrochemicals that were still dangerous. While the intention behind GE foods might have been good, many (including us) argue that that effort has gone utterly awry. In fact, today we are in much the same situation as our parents and grandparents were in when Rachel Carson was writing her book. In fact, we might be in a worse situation.

There is, of course, plenty of evidence that we got rid of the *worst* offenders in chemical fertilizers, pesticides, herbicides, and fungicides from the 1970s. Still, today we are locked in an escalating arms race of chemical pesticide warfare that is pushing us toward a predicament for our environment, our health, and the health of our kids. Genetic engineering technologies *did* initially reduce the overall need for very toxic pesticides, but the need for more and more pesticides (particularly herbicides) has grown exponentially since then *because of genetic engineering technologies*. On top of that, because of genetic engineering, we are now eating foods that have been turned into insecticides in their own right! Although controversy remains, we believe exposure to many of the chemicals used in industrial agriculture today is harming the people who work in our fields to produce these foods, and these chemicals are also harming the end consumers who eat them. We are all getting exposed to, and ingesting, large quantities of pesticides. In the chapters of this book you will learn how even low levels of exposure to the most commonly used chemicals in agriculture today can lead to negative health effects.

Turning to the question of how "safe" our pesticide-rich production of food is brings us straight to the work of Brenda Eskenazi, a public health epidemiologist who studies children who live in agricultural areas in the Salinas Valley in California that are exposed to high levels of pesticides.[9]

Her work is not on GM foods, but it is on pesticides, so let's look at what Dr. Eskenazi has found in relation to the battalion of chemicals used on most crops today.

Eskenazi's work shows that children with chronic exposure to pesticides have higher rates of neurodevelopmental problems. Specifically, she suggests that repeated low-level exposure to organophosphate pesticides affects neurodevelopment and growth, especially in children who do not have the enzymes to metabolize them. She talks about the possibility that these chemicals inhibit brain acetylcholinesterase and downregulate certain brain receptors (acetylcholine receptors). Acetylcholine is the neurotransmitter responsible for motor neurons that control skeletal muscles, and also for regulation of attention, arousal, learning, and memory.[10] Her work and the work of others, such as those involved in the Charge Study (at UC Davis), show that high exposure to organophosphates is associated with rates of neurological disorders in kids that are seven times the normal rate.[11]

Consider also the studies that show high rates of birth defects among migrant farmworkers or communities located near crops sprayed with methyl bromide—a fungicide commonly used on strawberries.[12] Consider studies that document how many pesticides are found in the blood of newborns and in breast milk in areas of high pesticide use, also showing that those exposed to organochlorines and pyrethroids, when compared to children from nonexposure areas, exhibit signs of delayed coordination and cognitive function.[13] We know that atrazine, a pesticide that was banned in Europe but is still used in the United States, causes endocrine disruption and, in adults, reproductive failure and cancer.[14] Birth defects are also associated with use of the pesticide chlorpyrifos, a chemical that the Obama administration's Environmental Protection Agency (EPA) recommended be banned but was quickly cleared for use in the Trump administration's EPA.[15] This is all before we get to the pesticide we (not Eskenazi or her colleagues) are most concerned with, Roundup—the most widely used pesticide today—and its active ingredient, glyphosate. All of these chemicals are used regularly on crops now and, despite regulations that aim to prevent harm, little is being done to limit exposures.

Eskenazi's work on the risks of pervasive long-term exposure to low or medium levels of the harshest chemicals among farmworkers should raise alarms. Children in agricultural areas are exposed to these chemicals through breast milk, pesticide drift, pesticides that get tracked into homes, pesticides that reside in dust, and, of course, foods that are eaten and have this residue *on* them or in *them* at the time of consumption.[16] So, if agrochemical industries' turn to biotechnology was intended to reduce the use of harsh chemicals in agriculture, it is fairly clear now that things have not worked out that way.

As homes are being built closer and closer to farmlands (or as more and more farmlands are converted into housing developments), the risks of exposure are expanding.[17] Harmful pesticides seep into groundwater, and researchers like Eskenazi signal a huge health epidemic that spills far beyond the farm. The results of their studies should be of concern not just to those who live in agricultural areas. When you consider that most of these chemicals *are being absorbed into the plants themselves* and subsequently eaten, the problem becomes much more geographically pervasive. We are concerned with the routes of exposure that are far from the farmlands. We are worried about the exposures coming from the water and milk we drink and the foods on our supermarket shelves. Before we get to these foods, though, let's first look at the problem of toxic exposures more widely and consider what regulatory agencies can (and cannot) do about them.

Other Toxic Chemical Exposures

Add to the list of multiple chemical exposures our children face today those that have nothing to do with our food production, such as PCBs, parabens, phthalates, styrenes, and petrochemical residues[18]—chemicals found in plastics and paper products that are used every day, in body care and cleaning products, in our water supply, and in the air we breathe. Sandra Steingraber, in *The Toxic Sandbox*, reminds us that even our most benign and banal activities can be filled with dangerous chemicals that are harmful to our children.

Indeed, foods are not the only way that people are exposed to toxic chemicals. Beth Greer, author of *Supernatural Home*, notes that many of these chemicals are used in common products such as food packaging and sunscreen. In fact, it is easy and simple for chemicals to enter the body and to accumulate over time. Tracey Woodruff, a UC San Francisco research epidemiologist who used to work for the EPA, found in a study of 268 pregnant women that nearly 100 percent who were randomly sampled tested positive for the presence in their blood of polychlorinated biphenyls, organochlorine pesticides, PFCs, phenols, PBDEs, phthalates, polycyclic aromatic hydrocarbons, and perchlorate. Exposure to chemicals during fetal development increases the risk of adverse health consequences exponentially, including risk of birth outcomes, childhood morbidity, and adult disease and mortality.[19] In many of these women, a whopping eighteen chemicals were found in their blood.[20]

The fact is that most of these chemicals get into the body by way of environmental exposure. Being in places where there are chemicals usually results one way or another in the chemicals getting inside the body. But many of the worst chemicals (including some Woodruff found in pregnant women) start out and are used in agriculture. The fact that so many chemicals show up in the bloodstream, urine, stool, and organs and that they tend to be stored in fat means, however, that the use of these chemicals is not just an agricultural concern. They are part of our ecosystem and part of our biology. We are living and breathing them via our air, water, and foods all the time. In fact, our kids are exposed to them even before they are born. As Woodruff and colleagues remind us, quoting a researcher at the National Cancer Institute, (echoing others) "Our babies are being born pre-polluted."[21] And if exposure to household and industrial chemicals is frightening, consider the fact that combinations of the effects of these chemicals *with* the pesticides that come from industrial agriculture have never been studied in a meaningful way.[22]

We are living in a chemical soup, but do we need to when it comes to our foods? Should we also have to worry about the toxicants that are in our foods that, quite literally, we are making our soup with? In this book, we are choosing not to focus on the larger chemical hurricane that surrounds us and our children. Rather, we focus on the source of our chemical exposures that is less well known and therefore less likely to be a current concern for many of us. That is, the toxic chemicals that come from our industrialized food production system. We are specifically interested in the pesticides that were introduced and have grown exponentially in use since the 1990s, when we started growing and selling *crops that were designed to be used with them* (or, really, to be *turned into them*) through genetic modification. Finding the delicate balance between protecting crops, on the one hand, and protecting humans, on the other, is one that has vexed agribusiness industries for years. It has also turned many scientists and parents, unwittingly, into political activists.

We cannot discuss the rise in use of pesticides and toxic chemicals in industrialized food production without also discussing the use of GM technologies to grow our foods. Not surprisingly, the most important concerns about these technologies are the most controversial. Many questions have aroused this controversy. First, are genetic modification technologies actually *increasing* instead of decreasing the amount of toxic chemicals that are being used in crop production? Second, are the genetically engineered foods that are grown with these pesticides, and are now in plentiful supply, studied sufficiently enough to know whether or not they are themselves dangerous to humans, and particularly to children? Third, are the agrochemicals associated with GM food production actually toxic and if so *how toxic* (i.e., *at what levels* are they toxic)?

Depending on how we answer the above questions, corollary questions arise as well: Are we witnessing an epidemic of dangerous exposure to the very things that have been putatively used to ensure a safe and reliable food supply? Is it GM crops or just the pesticides that come with them that we should be worried about? Are our children our "canaries in the coal mine" of our high-risk industrial food system? Are we in the midst of another *Silent Spring*? How did we get here and what can we do about it?

Responding to Jane Goodall's question in the epigraph of this chapter, "How could we have ever believed that it was a good idea to grow our food with poisons?" we could answer, "Easily." We collectively tend to believe in the United States in the dictum of better living through chemicals. We have historically solved many of our food supply problems by way of chemistry and industrial models of production. It has made us, and many corporations that have monopolies on our food systems, very rich! We also generally believed and continue to believe that the food industries are working with our best interests in mind, or that there are regulatory agencies that will protect us if they are not. And yet, we now know that many of the chemicals we use to safeguard our food production are not without harm, and in fact are quite toxic. In fact, not only do we now use poisons to grow our food, but also we have turned much of our food into what many would consider a form of poison in and of itself. How did this happen? Who is watching the henhouse?

Regulation as a Public Good

The concerns raised by environmental health scholars are similar to those raised by researchers looking at pesticides. Most people would be surprised, however, to learn there is a shocking lack of rigorous testing and regulation of chemicals in the United States. One would expect our food supply to be well regulated, but in far too many cases the three federal government agencies that bear responsibility for some aspect of food safety have not been exercising adequate oversight. These agencies are the FDA, the USDA (US Department of Agriculture), and the EPA.

The FDA has been granted the major role, and it is supposed to be exercising great precaution. According to the stipulations of the Food, Drug, and Cosmetic Act, this agency must ensure that all new additives to our food that do not have a safe history of use prior to 1958 are demonstrated to be safe via standard scientific testing before they're allowed on the market. In cases where sufficient technical evidence of safety has already been produced, and this evidence is well-recognized among experts, the new additive can be deemed to be "generally recognized as safe" (GRAS), and the manufacturer is not required to produce additional evidence.

But these precautionary safeguards have been violated when it comes to genetically engineered foods. As the public interest attorney Steven Druker has revealed in his book, *Altered Genes, Twisted Truth*, even though the FDA has acknowledged that the various pieces of DNA inserted into genetically engineered organisms are within the purview of these laws, it has claimed they are exempt from testing because they are GRAS—despite the fact its own files demonstrate the agency knew that neither of the requirements for GRAS status had been satisfied. Druker argues that although (1) the FDA's own experts concluded that GM foods pose abnormal risks and need to be tested, (2) the agency also knew that a significant number of experts outside the agency also believed that safety testing is needed, and (3) the agency additionally knew that no technical evidence of safety had been generated, it covered up these facts and falsely proclaimed that the conditions for GRAS had been satisfied. Accordingly, Druker states that the FDA allowed GM foods to come to market without requiring any testing whatsoever.[23] GM foods that are pesticides or PIP (plant-incorporated protectant) are regulated by the EPA.

The USDA, the oldest of the three institutions, established in 1862, also regulates agrochemicals and the ways that farmers grow crops or raise livestock and poultry. However, their main concern in this regard is in relation to new technologies or chemicals jeopardizing existing animal and farm resources. They do not regulate agriculturally used chemicals in relation to their toxicity to humans. Nor do they regulate or test the foods themselves (once they have left the farm, so to speak).

Finally, the EPA was established in 1970 with a more general and loosely defined responsibility to protect human health and the environment, based on monitoring, standard setting, and enforcement. In 1976, Congress passed the Toxic Substances Control Act, which gave the EPA full power to control chemicals that posed a health risk to humans and the environment. But have they?

The EPA's task has been to monitor the nearly 100,000 chemicals produced in or imported into the United States. Of these 100,000 chemicals, the EPA has only taken action to reduce the risk of over 3,600 chemicals, and it has banned or limited the production or use of *only 5*. It has not actually regulated a single chemical in the United States since the mid-1980s. Keep in mind, the EPA is the same agency responsible for determining the safe limits of pesticide residues in plants that are produced for human consumption.

On top of all this, the EPA's central stance on regulation is that chemicals are safe until proven otherwise. However, just how it determines this "safe" level is surprising. To determine maximum levels of exposure for certain chemicals, the EPA samples the concentrations of a chemical in the population. In other words, the EPA does *not* conduct rigorous research on the effects of chemicals; rather, it surveys the population and figures out how much is already present with the *assumption* that that amount is safe. This sets a range for an acceptable amount.

The EPA also does rigorous searches of the available research literature on toxicity from chemicals. The obvious flaws in this logic are twofold: First, adverse health effects are often not immediate or acute, but rather are long term before they develop as chronic problems. It is difficult to decipher exact causes of environmentally induced health effects, especially if they take a long time to develop. Chronic low levels of chemicals can accumulate in the body over time, and create long-term health effects such as cancer, but these are not going to be seen for decades.[24] Thus, "safe levels" are likely to be inaccurate and the use of dangerous chemicals might persist for many decades because toxicity is not yet apparent. This is in addition to the complications around using studies of chemical toxicities, which we will hear more about later.

Second, in regard to the EPA's use of scientific studies when it comes to foods, it follows the pattern of the FDA. Many studies on chemicals in foods are focused on establishing equivalence with existing foods, showing that they are no more dangerous than foods already in circulation. Thus, most foods do not fall under the scrutiny of the EPA, just as they don't under the FDA. The EPA does, however, exercise regulatory power over the use of foods that have *become* pesticides in and of themselves (such as some GM foods) because it is charged with regulating pesticides. However, the EPA has never actually curtailed use of these pesticide foods.

Finally, studies on chemical toxicities that are done in animals are almost exclusively done by the industries that produce and sell them, raising questions about bias and validity that are seldom heard at any of these regulatory agencies. The EPA accepts standards set by chemical companies that are based on their own research of "safe levels" or what are called "no observed adverse effect levels" (NOAELs). These levels are based on exposure tests on animals or humans, comparing biologically or statistically significant changes between test and control groups for alteration of morphology, functional capacity, growth, development, or life span. The EPA takes into account a variety of different measures of safe levels, which can vary from state to state, including no significant risk levels (NSRLs), maximum allowable dose levels (MADLs), and chronic reference dose levels (cRfD), depending on what type of disorder or toxicity one is looking at.

What all this adds up to is that despite the fact that many of these chemicals have been assigned "safe levels" of exposure and are on the market for use in our homes, schools, and businesses, they are often adjusted later, after reports begin to trickle in about possible effects or about exposure-related effects that are below these safe levels. Even when safety levels are set, often these minimal regulations are only made by the EPA in response to complaints, lawsuits, and hard-fought advocacy work of public interest organizations, rather than because the EPA is proactive and, on its own, does research to test safety.

Shifting the burden of proof of safety to industries has resulted in outcomes that should have been expected; industries are not very good at policing themselves.[25] And, it turns out, neither is the EPA, FDA, or USDA very good at protecting us. The coordination between industry, health researchers, and government regulation in the area of agrochemicals used in food production is abysmal. So, if we are quite literally surrounded by and bathing in—and entirely unable to escape from—the chemical hurricane that has arrived with the scientific engineering of our food supply, what sort of science, what kind of regulation, and what sort of medicine should we practice to deal with this?

To answer this question, we first need to explore what these poisons are and how exactly they impact our health. It turns out that answering these questions is not so easy. After all, not *everyone* who eats these foods gets sick, or at least not right away. In fact, some people never do, and this has created huge skepticism among many. As we have seen (and will continue to explore in this book), food industries and agribusinesses have spent a good deal of time assuring us that these foods and the chemicals we use to grow these foods are safe. Finally, again, the USDA, the EPA, and the FDA are not telling us that these crops are dangerous. Is it possible, however, that in our effort to ensure a sufficient food supply and profit margin for our farming communities we have had the wool pulled over our collective eyes when it comes to food safety?

Leaving aside the issues of meat, poultry, and dairy that are full of antibiotics and hormones (and that eat grain and grass crops that are genetically modified), what are these crops we are so worried about? The genetic engineering technologies that are of particular concern to food-focused medicine and to us are twofold. First is the genetic engineering of crops so that they are resistant to the herbicide Roundup, referred to as "Roundup Ready crops." These crops are specifically modified genetically to withstand death from glyphosate. That is, they are designed to enable use of Roundup. The second is the genetic engineering of crops so they contain the natural insecticide *Bacillus thuringiensis* toxin (Bt toxin). Bt is almost always used in conjunction with Roundup Ready genetic modifications. Plants modified with Bt are designed to kill pests trying to eat them; in fact, the plants themselves are turned into insecticides. No matter what part of the plant is eaten by a pest, it will kill the insect. Again, arguments for and against the safety of these genetic engineering technologies in food crops are controversial on both sides.[26]

When you consider that most of the Roundup Ready crops, including soy, corn, canola, alfalfa, cotton, sugar beets, apples, potatoes, and, soon, wheat (although experimental forms of genetically modified wheat do exist), are getting drenched in glyphosate and other herbicides as a normal part of their agricultural production, questions about how many of these chemicals are ending up in the foods we eat, and in the environment, naturally follow.

Prior to GM crops, farmers could not spray herbicides on the crops themselves, because the herbicides killed the food crops along with the weeds. Farmers sprayed the *soil* prior to planting. With the advent of Roundup Ready crops (and now, new GM crops that are resistant to stronger, more toxic herbicides), for the first time, farmers are able to spray the food itself—repeatedly—meaning a vastly increased amount of herbicides has entered directly into our food supply in just the past two decades.[27]

When you further consider that many of these food crops are themselves also modified to act like pesticides against living organisms, questions about what exactly these foods are doing inside of our guts, and specifically to the microorganisms in our guts, naturally arise as well. When you consider that poultry and livestock are fed foods with these same genetic modifications, plus the large quantities of added herbicides that accompany them, then questions about the pervasive dissemination of these chemicals into the animals that we consume escalate quickly. Finally, when you consider that most processed foods—even baby formula and baby foods in most US grocery stores today—are made from these crops (especially soy and corn or their derivatives), then one begins to see the contours of our contemporary *Silent Spring*.

We will discuss more about these biotechnologies, and the chemicals they depend on, and we will learn more about the disputed science around them in chapter 11 (where we will dive deeper into the regulatory nuances, as well). For now, let's return to some examples of the clinical experiences arising from our *second Silent Spring*. Exactly how are these chemically dependent tactics for food production impacting the human body and specifically the health of our children? There is much less information about this topic, and virtually none available to clinicians. Even clinicians who are aware of these profound disruptions in the environment and in our food will have a hard time parsing the information and applying it to their clinical practices. This interface is challenging at best, daunting at worst. This lack of information is appalling considering the pervasiveness of genetically modified crops that saturate the food supply of Americans today.

CHAPTER FIVE

The Family Eating Modern Industrial Foods: Almost Everyone Is Sick

Our babies are being born pre-polluted.

SHARYLE PATTON, Director of the Commonweal Biomonitoring Resources Center[1]

Marilyn was a high-powered litigator who ran her own business and was married to a successful businessman. They lived a typical upper-middle-class life, with their share of challenges around work-family balance. But it had not always been this way. Marilyn described her family history as one in which "almost everyone was sick."

Her daughter, Carrie, was about eighteen months old when Marilyn first came to Dr. Perro for Carrie's chronic upper respiratory problems. Neither of Marilyn's two children were healthy back then, nor was she. Marilyn described it vividly. Carrie had a lot of sinus pain, big thick gunk clogging up her nose, and dark circles under her eyes. Her cheeks were dented in. She looked sick. She was an unhappy baby, crying all of the time. It was clear she was miserable.

When we asked how long Carrie had these problems, Marilyn went back to the beginning. At five weeks old Carrie was having a lot of gastrointestinal issues. Her poop was completely mucousy, and green. If you put a wipe into the diaper, you could pull up a six-inch string of mucus, which was not a good sign. She had chronic ear infections, and she could hardly breathe due to her stuffy nose; she was breathing through her mouth and, as a result, was coughing all the time. She couldn't sleep, and would cry all night long.

Carrie's first pediatrician, after prescribing multiple courses of antibiotics, diagnosed Carrie as having an allergy to milk protein. She advised Marilyn to adjust her own diet because Carrie, at that time, was being exclusively breastfed. Marilyn said she was really careful with what she ate: no milk, chocolate, butter. She would read labels to make sure she didn't eat anything with even the slightest bit of dairy in it. She said, "Carrie wasn't getting any of it. She started getting a little bit better. The poops got a little better, but she still had the congestion."

Marilyn realized early on that Carrie's problems fluctuated with her own diet. She was having . . . "I'll call them reactions because they are technically not allergies," she said. It was easy to regulate her diet at home, but when she went traveling out of town with the family and they would eat at restaurants, she'd eat foods that she didn't normally eat. She noticed that Carrie got sick soon after. "It would fluctuate with other foods I was eating like soy, nuts, bananas, canola oil . . . all of those things. I could tell how she was reacting especially around four or five in the morning." Twice while they were traveling she had to take Carrie to the emergency room, to urgent care, after she had been screaming all night long. "We went nine nights in a row with almost no sleep. Obviously she was suffering, but we were all suffering," Marilyn said.

Marilyn heard about Dr. Perro by way of another integrative physician she was working with for her own health challenges. The first thing Dr. Perro advised Marilyn to do was to switch to only organic foods. Marilyn said this was a big hurdle. Her husband was convinced these foods would cost too much, and he didn't believe they would make any difference. But Marilyn pushed it. "We have to try it even if it is only for a few weeks," she thought. So she did. And within a week she started noticing improvements. "The congestion . . . instead of being all gunked up, Carrie was just a little bit drippy. Her cheeks stopped having the dents and puffiness," she recalled. She said Carrie's eyes brightened up, and her language got better, her ear infections subsided. She figured Carrie's hearing had been impaired by all the infections and congestion, and when this cleared up all of a sudden her language "went from zero to sixty." She said, "I can't believe how fast it switched and she was just really progressing with language. Everything got better. She would sleep better; she would cry less. She would still cry around 5 a.m. or so, but instead of it being a horrifying scream like she was being attacked, it became just a little whiney cry. There was still something going on, but she was obviously feeling better."

Marilyn showed us pictures of her daughter at both two and three years old and the before and after comparison was remarkable. In the "after" photo, Carrie's eyes were bright, and she'd lost the puffiness. Her color was rosy instead of pasty. As far as Marilyn was concerned, the switch to organic foods made all the difference. She couldn't really explain it, but she was certain it mattered. She even tested this theory. After a few months, she let her daughter eat some foods that were not organic and her congestion came back almost instantly.

Like so many other kids Dr. Perro has treated, Carrie was one more child demonstrating the benefits of shifting to organic. Removing foods that she was sensitive to was the first step, but that alone was not enough. When she eliminated nonorganic foods, all the other symptoms went away. The clinical observation seemed to point to the possibility that nonorganic foods were doing something to trigger all these food sensitivities. They seemed to be the underlying culprits.

At around this time, Marilyn also brought her son, Jason, to see Dr. Perro. Jason, who was a few years older than Carrie, had the opposite problem. Her daughter would eat everything but was "reactive" to it. Her son would not eat *anything*. This, too, started when he was very little. He had a difficult time latching on for nursing. Marilyn also described her own feeling of being sick after his birth. She was extraordinarily tired and depressed. "All moms are tired after birth," she said, "but I felt like I was having a pity party. I wasn't even safe to drive. I was really struggling."

One of the symptoms Marilyn developed after the birth of her son was burning eyes. She initially assumed it was from sleep deprivation from struggling so much with her son. He just wouldn't eat. As she mentioned, she couldn't get him to latch on to her breast. She worked with lactation consultants, but that didn't help either. The whole time she was struggling with huge fatigue, and her eyes were getting worse. Then she began to have significant joint pain. She thought she might have arthritis.

Eventually, Marilyn went to a rheumatologist, and he told Marilyn to go off gluten, sugar, and dairy. She described her reaction honestly. "I burst into tears. I was like, 'Noooo, what'll I do if I can't eat gluten, sugar, or dairy?'" But, she did it. She went off them for a week and described being at a restaurant and seeing bread and thinking, "Well, I can have a little." She had two bites and was immediately in pain—nearly on the floor. Her symptoms returned with a vengeance: the horrible brain fog, pain in her joints, and the burning eyes. When she stayed off gluten, her symptoms were manageable. After multiple consultations, her doctor finally diagnosed her as having Sjogren's disorder, which is an autoimmune disorder in which the body attacks the moisture-producing glands, producing dry eyes, dry mouth, and fatigue.

Sjogren's disorder, also called Sjogren's syndrome, is mostly prevalent in women forty or older. It is not hereditary, though there is some speculation of a genetic correlation, and it might be related to rheumatic disease. Marilyn described her mouth as being so dry she couldn't get through the night without drinking a full glass of water. As it turns out, there isn't really a cure for Sjogren's in conventional medicine, although there are ways to suppress the symptoms. Treatments include eye drops for moisturizing the eyes, drugs to increase saliva, and methotrexate to suppress the immune system. For some people, a medicine used to treat malaria can also be effective in reducing Sjogren's symptoms. Marilyn said she didn't try any of these. For her, getting off the gluten made a huge difference, and she avoided the more serious drugs.[2]

Marilyn thought her health condition might have had something to do with her son's problems with food, too. Again, he was a poor eater from birth, she said. The comparison with her daughter was partly what helped Marilyn to recognize that he wasn't healthy. Her daughter was larger at birth, but she also ate well despite all her chronic health issues. Jason was small when he was born, and it was as if he never had an appetite for eating at all. The situation with Jason only got worse the older he got and the more they tried to introduce solid foods. "At five years old," she said, "he still had really severe feeding issues. Basically, he wouldn't eat. It is really hard to talk about." Marilyn's eyes began to tear up as she described her struggle. "It was as if he was terrified of foods. He only ate yogurt." She described a time when Jason was about one year old and she was preparing an apple, cutting it and peeling it and setting it on his tray, and he got excited about it. His face lit up like he couldn't wait to get it. But when he touched it and noticed it was wet, he recoiled, and refused to eat it. He would gag and vomit, and this was with everything.

Marilyn said that at a certain point, she sort of gave up. Of course, this led to him being underweight. But it also turned into problems with his emotions. He got very "rage-y," she said. He would get extremely moody and have tantrums every hour. She said she thought all this was related to the fact that he wasn't getting enough nourishment. He was probably cranky from being hungry all the time. His regular pediatricians kept telling her that her son was just a picky eater and that she should be stricter with him. She thought they really didn't get it. It was pathology, not an issue of preference.

When Marilyn started with Dr. Perro, she was able to explain the history of Jason's food issues with a depth that was remarkable. Dr. Perro already knew a lot about Marilyn's situation and her kids, having worked with Jason's younger sister, Carrie. So, Dr. Perro started Jason on several different homeopathic remedies, which seemed to help calm him down. But she also worked with Marilyn to figure out how to get more nutrients into the things he *would* eat. This included yogurt, and pretty much only yogurt. So, they devised a way to make yogurt shakes that contained added nutrients, supplements with vitamins, and, most important of all, probiotics (live bacteria and yeasts that, when consumed, offer various health benefits, including supporting the gut). Marilyn, however, was skeptical about a lot of these interventions, and it took a lot of convincing from Dr. Perro to try them out. Working to change Jason's diet was arduous because Marilyn was convinced he wouldn't go for any of the proposed solutions. Still, she gave it a try.

Marilyn said that Jason's health changed dramatically after the changes to his diet. He started growing. He started to talk about what foods he wanted, and even began to try eating new things. His rage-iness went away. Marilyn showed us before and after photos of her son, too. It was true—he looked sick in the "before" photo, and very malnourished. But Jason looked like a normal kid in the "after" one, with shiny hair and a big smile. His arms were still thin, but he looked more like a thin kid than like a malnourished one. Marilyn's own health improved dramatically as she modified her family's diet, and after taking homeopathic remedies for another six months, while staying off gluten, she actually got rid of her Sjogren's. In fact, when she went in for another antibody test at five months after diagnosis after having had the problem for years, there was no longer any evidence of the antibodies in her blood.

Marilyn and both of her kids had problems with their bodies' ability to eat and use food in a normal way. For Marilyn, the problem was related to sensitivity to gluten that, she believed, triggered Sjogren's. For her son, it was not clear what caused his inability to eat, but Marilyn guessed his digestive system was probably undeveloped. For her daughter, it was extraordinary sensitivity to *all* kinds of foods, starting with dairy. Getting Carrie off dairy and then eating nothing but organic foods seemed to have cleared up her health problems almost entirely. For all of them, changing their diets (each in different ways) made a huge difference in their health.

As far as Marilyn was concerned, the most important treatment for all of their ailments was food—figuring out the right foods to eat that would enable their bodies to thrive as opposed to inducing reactions. This involved a combination of eliminating things they had a reaction to but also feeding their bodies foods that they could use, foods that were not exacerbating their already overtaxed immune systems; in other words, foods that would enable their guts to heal. Dealing with sensitivity issues got easier and easier the healthier all of their guts became. The more they stayed on organic foods, the healthier they got, and eventually they were even able to eat the foods they had once been sensitive to, with no bad reactions. Marilyn felt that transitioning to organic and cutting out all GM foods was the big step that changed everything for all of them. It was as if they were all able to process or eliminate the toxicants from their systems because their digestive systems, and their entire gastrointestinal tracts, were finally doing their jobs right.

It would be oversimplistic to attribute their recoveries to just one factor: switching to organic foods. There are many factors that played into the radical health changes they experienced. Some part of Marilyn's problems might have been related to her genetic makeup, and this also might have been at play with the children through epigenetics—heritable changes between parent and child in the way genes are expressed. If Marilyn was exposed to too many plastics, for instance, or heavy metals or even pesticides *on* or *in* her food while she was pregnant with her children, those exposures could have created alterations in the way her genes were being switched on and off. These changes in the expression of genetics could have been inherited by her children, making for significant health problems.

Part of Marilyn's health problems might have been augmented by the emotional stress of new motherhood and the challenge of taking care of sick kids who were struggling with food. Cortisol levels change with stress and these, too, can lead to chronic inflammation in the body. Still, the entire family was impacted, and able to correct many of the problems they had, by changing *what they were eating*, period. Treating Marilyn's kids required helping Marilyn comprehend a rather colossal shift in her own attitude about food and health. She eventually came to see how problems with complex causal pathways could be funneled into basic and easy-to-implement solutions. At first, Marilyn was skeptical about many of the remedies and approaches Dr. Perro advised, despite the fact that she saw radical improvements in her own health and her children's just by changing their diets. She was not initially easily convinced that these simple remedies would work or that she would be able to deploy these remedies with her children. But she was able, and they did work.

From the perspective of a clinician, approaches to disorders like Marilyn's and her children's require an ability to hold many different causal chains in the mix and to shift back and forth between the effects and the causes, in a cyclical manner. While complex system malfunctions are involved in each different case, treatments can be very straightforward and simple, starting with food. It makes sense that we would see different impacts of exposure to unhealthy foods because so many factors are at play: genetics, epigenetics, age at exposure, the variety of exposure, and, most important of all, different toxic load capacities from person to person. Overuse of antibiotics in the normal routines of medical care might play a role here. Socioeconomic status plays into this, too, and not just because access to healthy food is often correlated with social class. Kids from wealthy families are often eating processed foods and exposed to multiple chemicals in their environments (although kids living in lower-income neighborhoods tend to be at greater risk for a significant array of chemical exposures and also tend to have less available healthy food).

Genetically modified foods, interestingly, are pervasive in the United States across socioeconomic classes and geography. Because of their ubiquity across socioeconomic levels, they can be an equalizer in an otherwise unequal society. Wealthy, middle-income, and low- or no-income families all eat GM foods. The same is not true of organic foods, of course, which are currently mostly only available to wealthy or middle-class communities. Even within families across the spectrum, however, we see differences in each individual's ability to respond to toxicants that come from foods.

Just as we see different abilities in many things, from sports to mathematics, different capacities to process and manage toxic exposures vary. We're not all built the same and we're not all exposed to the same things, and therefore we don't process things the same way or at the same rates. This is why mothers frequently talk about how one child who ate the same foods as another seems to be perfectly healthy while a second child has incredible food issues, from allergies and sensitivities to other problems with eating. Marilyn's family was a good example of this, even though both children had some issues.

To put it more simply: Not *all* people will get sick from eating unhealthy foods at the same rate. This does not mean, however, we should assume that those foods are therefore healthy. Just because some kids can eat lots of junk food and not get sick for a long time does not mean they are healthy. They might, in fact, be doing damage to their guts and other organs (especially the liver) without realizing it. Once they reach their toxic load limits, they might begin to show signs of illness. As we will go into later in chapter 12, liver problems are now showing up in kids at escalating rates.[3] Sometimes this damage goes undetected for a long time, much like the variable effects on the liver from alcohol consumption among adults. For other kids who start out with some disadvantages in relation to their body's ability to handle toxic things (including antibiotics, chemicals, and pesticides), their path to sickness might be quite short.

Thinking about food as a source of toxicity for our children portends the need for an *ecosystems approach* to clinical care. The health of the gut is a huge component of overall health, and our gut health is largely related to what we eat (and, of course, it also has to do with other things, such as birth, genetics, and environment). If the food we are eating is not nutritious, or worse, if it is itself contaminated by things our guts cannot handle, we get sick.

Forward-thinking scientists and physicians are advancing several theories about how all this works. Marilyn's story makes more sense when we look more deeply at some of the new thinking about the microbiome, dysbiosis, and leaky gut. We'll look at these in the next chapter.

CHAPTER SIX

The Gut Microbiome, Symbiosis, and Dysbiosis

Studies are finding that our bacteria (or lack thereof) can be linked to or associated with: obesity, malnutrition, heart disease, diabetes, celiac disease, eczema, asthma, multiple sclerosis, colitis, some cancers, and even autism.

THE AMERICAN MICROBIOME INSTITUTE[1]

Patients like Marilyn and her kids have to work hard to find doctors who will put together the pieces of their stories and work collaboratively with them to figure out how to resolve their health issues. This is often in addition to working against opposition to these efforts from their family members, friends, workmates, and even from some of their regular doctors who don't take a food-centered approach. Food-related disorders (not including allergies) could take a long time to show up, and the causal links are not always immediately visible. Despite the fact that food should be seen as the most important ingredient in our health and our disorders, mainstream medical science does not always offer clear and coherent maps of the causal pathways when it comes to food that might be invisibly toxic.

Aside from the few known disorders directly caused by foods, such as celiac disease, diabetes, and allergies or intolerances, up until a few years ago we had surprisingly scant research on the relationships between foods and chronic diseases, and almost nothing on digestive system health and chronic diseases. There were a few pioneering physicians who explored nutritional therapies in psychiatry[2] and there were nutritionists (who were often not utilized in mainstream medicine). This lack of research is partly because of the problems we mentioned before: a preference for drug approaches, a lack of funding for food-based therapies, and the difficulty of conducting feeding study clinical trials.

Things are changing in biomedical science today. One of the most promising new areas of research that might point to the causal paths between food and health disorders is research that focuses on the gut microbiome. Since the gut is the key organ involved in turning food into its nutritional components, it makes sense for us to start there.

What is new research telling us about the gut microbiome? The microbiome (officially named by scientists around 2001) is defined as the collection of microorganisms—a multitude of roughly 3 billion bacterial communities—that make up the exterior and interior lining of the human body.[3] It turns out that humans are significantly bacterial in composition. Furthermore, research is showing that bacteria are not the only communities that coinhabit, or compose, the human. There are also communities of viruses (the virome) as well as fungi (mycobiome). We call these, collectively, the *microbiome*.

What new research points to is the idea that instead of thinking of humans in terms of our own genetics and cellular composition, we need to think of humans as collections of many bacterial species, each with specific collections of genes and cells. Recent measures have found a 1:1 ratio of microorganisms to human cells.[4] And, while these bacteria as well as other microbes live on our skin, and on the surface of our eyes, in our nasal passages, and in all of our orifices, among their most populous locations is in our digestive tract, otherwise known as our guts—which begins with the mouth and concentrates in the stomach, the intestines, and finally the colon.

Different sections of the digestive tract tend to have different colonies of microbes, although some can move undesirably from one section to another. Our mouths have some similar and some different microbes than our stomachs and our colons. Health problems can arise when colonies that belong only in one region migrate to another, where they wreak havoc on other microbes that prefer to live there. Gut microbiomes are not the same from population to population. They can differ in composition based on many things, including geography, food environments, genetics, and climate. There is new research on microbiome composition across populations and within families. Though these tests do not present perfect reflections of what is actually in the gut, they show that microbial communities are more likely to be shared between parents and children rather than across geographic regions, but these communities can even differ within geographic regions. We know that environment (including diet and even the family dog) plays a large role in configuring microbiome composition.[5]

Thus, it is impossible to define a universal healthy microbiome in terms of a defined population of microbes. Again, "normal" gut populations can vary from individual to individual even within geographically similar populations; nevertheless, there are some similarities across populations. Scientists are starting to trace some important patterns in microbe colonies of the gut that appear to produce similar kinds of symptoms, or health, across geographic and individual differences, as we'll see in a moment. What comes out of all this research is that ultimately having a *healthy* microbiome is extremely important to optimal health.[6]

The important fact to know about the microbiome is that it is *alterable*. This is one of the most unique and powerful things about it—we can influence the composition of the microbiome by what we eat. Although certain characteristics of the microbiome appear to be laid down at birth (or before), within an individual, the microbiome can shift with changes in age, diet, geographical location, and intake of food supplements and drugs. The microbiome is a dynamic human organ, influencing alterations in gene expression as well. From this perspective, making changes to diet—the least invasive form of medicine there is, and arguably the least expensive—might prove to be an important means of therapy.

Researchers suspect that by early childhood (most say by the age of two or three), the microbiome of most healthy children is established—that is, in a healthy gut, the baseline population of microbial colonies is in place.[7] It starts to be developed at, or perhaps before, birth, and certainly grows rapidly after delivery in the infant, starting with acquisition of the mother's vaginal microbiome as it passes through the birth canal.[8] There is a rich microbial community in breast milk as well. Once established, the microbiome is key to instructing the thymus (the gland in the neck that produces T cells for the immune system) in how to regulate and develop innate immunity. The microbiome also plays an important role in detoxification, prior to the work the liver does, by deciphering which elements of our food are micronutrients and which need to be extruded as waste. Two of the most important things the bacteria of our gut do are repair the intestinal lining and, as mentioned, produce key vitamins and amino acids. This is the part of digestion that we are most interested in, or what is most relevant to figuring out the relationships between chronic diseases, pesticide exposure, and food-focused medicine. What happens when the gut microbiome is poorly developed, or when it is severely impacted and compromised, undermining the colonies of microbes that are needed for all of these physiological processes? To explore this, let's look for a minute at a theory of symbiosis.

Symbiosis and Dysbiosis

Thinking about health through the lens of the microbiome helps us think about human health in relation to the health of our ecosystem. Mary Roach, in her book *Gulp: Adventures on the Alimentary Canal*, talks about how the human body is like a donut.[9] The lining of our inner digestive canal is contiguous with the external lining of our body, the skin, and thus both are exposed to the environment in one way or another. Another way of saying this is: By way of the microbiome, we are in direct or indirect contact with—meaning we are indivisibly part of—the external environment in which we live. Microbes form a porous and lively layer between the human body and the world outside of it, but we can think of it as less of a boundary and more of a communication system. In many ways, the microbiome is its own ecosystem, with metabolic and physiological networks we are just now learning about, but the microbiome also lives in a larger ecosystem—it is a key translational medium between internal and external environment. It reflects, in our bodies, much of what occurs in the wider world.

It is worth thinking about how we might need to revise our very notion of the human body, or even perhaps what it means to be human, with the microbiome in mind. We are *not* inert or individual. Rather, we are permeable and we are multiple. Anthropologists like to call humans "multispecies beings," or, what Michael Pollan calls, "superorganisms."[10] Our microbes are in some sense *us*. Thus, it makes sense that we need to think about what kind of environment we are part of. Our cells are quite literally interacting with our outer world all the time.

Symbiosis is a good word to describe the best possible relationship between microbiomes and their human hosts (or should we say humans and their microbial hosts?). Symbiosis refers to the condition that arises from harmonious relationships between organisms that live together. Mutualism or commensalism is implied in this use of the term in the sense that the relationships involve exchanges of nutrients and by-products that enable mutual survival. At optimal functioning, we live symbiotically with our microbes in the sense that we house and feed them, but they also house and feed us. In many ways, it would be truest to say that we humans are mere temporary repositories for the teeming, complex, and very successful colonies of bacteria that live through us. It thus matters immensely not only how we ensure that our microbiome is established firmly, but that it remains healthy. In a word, it matters what we feed our microbiome—which has a great deal to do with what we "feed" our environment.

The influential evolutionary biologist, Lynn Margulis, wrote eloquently about how human evolution could only have happened by way of symbiotic relations between cellular entities. She argued that our own cellular organelles—mitochondria—were once independent, free-living bacteria. Their current cohabitation in human cells was a product of natural selection that favored symbiotic existence—that is, a system that favored mutual survival rather than survival of only the fittest in a zero sum game. Her discussions of the Gaia hypothesis that treats symbiosis as a core principle of our ecosystem are now shifting our conversations about not only human survival but also planetary survival.[11]

How might symbiosis help us make sense of gut health and toxic foods? As we've said, gut microbiota are the key components of the living architecture of the gut. Microbes provision the gut, and thus the human, with nutrients. Humans also provision their bacteria with nutrients (even by way of food), as we will see. It is even more complicated, however. Researchers are finding that these bacteria communicate with one another via something called *quorum sensing*. Quorum sensing is what happens when a colony of bacteria gets to be a certain size and the individual bacteria are able to perform different and stronger actions than they could in a less dense (less populous) community, again suggesting a type of symbiosis achieved through communication by way of "signaling molecules." These micro and group-based communication systems turn out to be important in efforts to treat kids who have chronic diseases, as we will see, since getting gut health right is in many cases more about finding the right balance than it is about killing enemies or keeping out intruders. Models of health based on coevolution and symbiosis of our multispecies being are key to dealing with chronic disorders.

When gut bacteria are disrupted—and they can be disrupted by many things—all or some of these functions might go awry. Colonies of bacteria can mobilize or communicate with one another to protect themselves and the host, or they can be harmful. Chronic disorders can start here. For instance, a healthy gut means a healthy balance of microorganisms, so one kind of gut disruption is when this balance is undermined: when too many of one kind of bacteria proliferate and too many of another bacteria decline. This imbalance is called *dysbiosis*, which can mean a number of things: missing microbes, an overproliferation of harmful bacteria, and a reduction or elimination of helpful bacteria, for example.[12]

This process of disruption of gut microbes can start even before food is eaten, and even before birth. As we mentioned, a pregnant mother's *own* dysbiosis, which can be caused by use of antibiotics or a variety of other factors (including genetics, smoking, and exposure to chemicals, to name a few) can also affect the child through epigenetic changes in the mother that are inherited by the child.[13] Research now shows that during the last month of the intrauterine period, the fetus becomes colonized by microbes, inside the womb.[14] The birth process, as previously mentioned, also affects the child's microbiome. Newborns who are delivered by Caesarean section miss out on the transmission of important bacteria lining the mother's birth canal.[15] The fact that nearly one-third of American births are Caesarean section makes the clinical implications of this problem far-reaching. Although many practitioners advise rubbing the mother's vaginal secretions on the newborn to facilitate bacterial transmission by imitating passage through the birth canal, clinical guidelines are being debated about this. Beyond birth, though, the microbiome can be impacted early on. Children who are put on antibiotics as infants, like Trevor, Georgia's son who had ulcerative colitis, are at a disadvantage in developing a healthy microbiome, as are children who are fed antibiotics through mother's breast milk.[16]

Despite the fact that research on food and the microbiome is just starting to take off, there is already a growing amount of research on the relationships between the microbiome and general health, based on studies in animal populations. There is still little research on humans. Why is this the case? Part of the reason for the limited number of studies in humans is the nature of the research itself. In studies with laboratory animals, researchers are able to make microbiome changes by using procedures that cannot be used in humans, such as surgically implanting colonies or raising animals that start out as microbially known (that is, not infected with those bacteria that are being studied), such as gnotobiotic mice. Studies on humans must test for the composition of gut bacteria by using fecal genetic tests, which are currently used by many integrative practitioners, but they are seldom covered by health insurance. Still, we do know a lot from animal studies, and our repertoire of knowledge about how foods can feed our microbial populations in our guts is growing every day.

We could pause for a moment and ask a few questions about the notion of symbiosis. If our internal guts are influenced by external bacterial environments, then why shouldn't we see food as the diplomat, the chief negotiator, between these worlds? Are our food ecosystems interdependent and mutually benefitting symbiotic systems that extend from the outside (how we produce food) to the inside (to our gut microbiota)? Shouldn't we see food, in fact, as the key negotiator in sustaining healthy cohabitation of many species in our food environments and healthy microbial species in our guts? We think so, and we think this effort to explore symbiosis can also help explain why foods that are not nutritious (or, worse, are toxic) can have a huge impact on gut health. Later, we will also look at the way that healthy soils, made by healthy microbes and other critters, are needed to make healthy food. For now, let's stay with the gut a little longer to explore what we are learning about food and gut health from animal studies.

Unhealthy Guts and Diseases

Based largely on animal studies, there is a growing body of knowledge associating gut dysbiosis and specific diseases. For instance, studies suggest relationships between missing microbes and major health disorders, such as asthma, autism, multiple sclerosis, and diabetes.[17] B. Brett Finlay, one of the leading scientists on the microbiome, notes that dysbiosis is associated with the following diseases: obesity, metabolic syndrome, nonalcoholic steatohepatitis, inflammatory bowel disease (Crohn's disease, ulcerative colitis, pouchitis), irritable bowel syndrome and functional bowel disorders, atherosclerosis, Type 1 diabetes, autism, allergy, asthma, and celiac disease.[18] In his book *Let Them Eat Dirt*, cowritten with Marie-Claire Arrieta, Finlay argues that children need to be exposed to environments plentiful in bacteria during childhood in order to develop a healthy microbiome. To this advice, we would add the footnote: Let them eat dirt that is not full of toxic chemicals.

There are other studies suggesting compromises in the microbiome can result in depression, anxiety, ADHD, chronic fatigue, Type 2 diabetes, and colon cancer.[19] Although some studies merely point to correlations between the presence or absence of certain gut microbes and these disorders, there are also studies that show clear pathways between microbial gut health and brain health.[20] Some research has also shown that altering the gut microbiome of mice can alter metabolism in ways that lead to obesity,[21] and that these might be involved in epigenetic processes involved in passing on this problem generationally, as we will see.[22]

Mechanisms that explain the relationship between gut health and overall health as a balance also point to some system dysfunctions that tie the two together. The microbiome is intimately linked to proper functioning of the immune system, producing or suppressing inflammatory responses, and is therefore tied to autoimmune disorders, such as some of the diseases previously mentioned.[23] One study showed that adults with allergies, especially to nuts and seasonal pollen, have low diversity, reduced *Clostridiales* bacteria, and increased *Bacteroidales* bacteria in their gut.[24] Other research shows that patients with multiple sclerosis (an autoimmune disorder) have distinct microbiota profiles, also suggesting pathogenesis tied to dysbiosis.[25] Martin Blaser, in his book *Missing Microbes*, argues that overuse of antibiotics and other medical interventions that compromise gut health contribute to the rise of many chronic diseases. Specifically, he argues that *Helicobacter pylori* (*H. pylori*) has been associated with gastric ulcers, but because these parasitic microbes have evolved symbiotically with humans, they also confer health benefits to humans, especially in relation to healthy immune system function. He points to links between autoimmunity and healthy gut microbiomes, suggesting that people without these key bacteria might be at greater risk of autoimmune diseases.

Patients with chronic and intractable infections of *Clostridium difficile* (*C. difficile*), a normally harmless inhabitant of the gut that can become an opportunistic microbial pathogen in the guts of patients on antibiotics (and especially potent broad-spectrum antibiotics), are now thought to be treatable with fecal transplants. These transplants aim to restore healthy bacterial colonies to the microbiome not only so that harmful ones are minimized but also so that these helpful bacteria can do whatever it is they are doing (including producing micronutrients that humans need). The fact that we know that antibiotics can be very harmful to microbiome health is a point to keep in mind as we look at pesticides, later on.[26]

With the knowledge we have about the relationships between gut health and overall health, we are learning more each day about the relationships between specific *foods* and gut health. As we mentioned, once the microbiome is established, the microbes that live there on a quasi-permanent basis are fed or starved, nurtured or damaged by what we do, not by what we were born with. It makes sense that the health of our microbiota depends largely on what we put into the gut. Studies on the resiliency of the gut, exploring how it might be able to repair itself or recolonize in new ways that create new steady states post disease, are still being done. Research on the role of specific foods in relation to these activities of the microbiome is key here.

Justin and Erica Sonnenburg, molecular biologists and immunologists at Stanford University, offer important insights about what foods help nurture a healthy microbiome in their book, *The Good Gut*. Their laboratory research shows that microbes lining the gut like to eat indigestible fiber.[27] The fiber that cannot be digested into simple sugars finds its way into the lining of the intestines, where it sits, forming a protective layer on top of the mucosal layer, which, in turn, forms a protective layer on top of the epithelium (with its cilia-lined villi). A typical American diet lacks this fiber and instead is full of processed simple sugars that are digested quickly and early, before they get to the small intestine. Without this fiber in the small intestine, the microbes eat the mucus layer of the intestinal epithelium, compromising its function by thinning out the cilia layer. Essentially, the thickness of the layer is indicative of a healthy diet and satisfied microbes. Individuals with gastrointestinal tract problems like irritable bowel syndrome (IBS) have a much reduced mucus layer. In fact, some researchers suggest microbes might themselves be *a source of* the mucus layer and its associated metabolites.[28]

Peter Turnbaugh, a microbiologist at UC San Francisco, and Lawrence David, a microbiologist at Duke, have shown that our microbiomes can change rapidly even with short-term dietary change. Specifically, eating meat versus a plant-based diet over only two days resulted in dramatic changes in microbial populations in mice. The mice fed meat diets showed increased growth of microbes that are capable of triggering inflammatory bowel disease. Plant products altered the microbial community in a different way, by creating more fiber to support the epithelial layer of the gut. Specifically, carnivore diets promote the growth of bile-tolerant bacteria and decrease the level of firmicutes (bacteria) that metabolize dietary plant polysaccharides (carbohydrates).[29] Peter Turnbaugh's laboratory has shown that diet is by far the largest determinant and consistently resets and shapes the microbiome's composition over the short term and the long term,[30] but beyond this, we still don't know much about how different kinds of food production might result in different microbial sustenance or harm.

Turnbaugh has also been investigating the links between microbial composition and obesity. In studies of mice, he found that those with a higher proportion of firmicutes to bacteriodetes (more than the normal proportion, which is roughly 60:40 percent) are more likely to become obese.[31] We don't know for sure whether these microbiome differences are mostly a consequence of biological factors in the human populations (i.e., genetics or epigenetics) or a consequence of different food environments, or all of these, but there are reasons to think they are related primarily to food.

Understanding the huge variety of bacterial populations is a gigantic task. How microchanges in the gut are sustained, and their long-term impacts on health, especially with persistent dietary habits, is just beginning to be understood. These studies are already opening up space for inquiry about food environments and positive health outcomes in important new ways, but they are also forcing us to ask questions about how we impact gut health in negative ways as well, specifically by creating dysbiosis. If symbiosis is a healthy and mutually beneficial relationship of cohabitation, dysbiosis means the opposite: an unhealthy and destructive relationship of cohabitation. So, what are some known causes of dysbiosis?

Causes of Dysbiosis

As mentioned, we know that antibiotics can change the composition of the microbiome, leading to dysbiosis. Specifically, to restate, many antibiotics contribute to the overflourishing of opportunistic bacteria (including *C. difficile*, for example) to levels that are harmful. Antibiotics are also associated with the decrease of other beneficial bacteria that are needed for health, such as *Lactobacilli* and *Bifidobacteria*. Probiotics that contain the latter, in fact, are now recommended routinely to patients who have been on antibiotics, even for short-term use of antibiotics, in the hopes of restoring healthy microbes in their gut.[32]

Here is where our concern with food production becomes important. Antibiotics can enter our bodies not just through prescription medication or deliberate sanitation measures. They can also enter our guts unintentionally by way of our foods. Because of food production procedures such as universally treating livestock and poultry with antibiotics (to treat disease or to promote the animal's growth), we are saturating sectors of our food supply with antibiotics. This problem is not simply one of giving antibiotics to unwitting consumers; it also accelerates antibiotic resistance. The Institute of Medicine of The National Academies Food and Nutrition Board notes: "Extensive antibiotic use in the modern livestock farm exerts a selective pressure for antibiotic resistance that spreads beyond the farm to the ecosystem at large and eventually to the human microbiome."[33]

Some studies now show that common detergent-like food additives, such as lecithin, daten, CMC, and polysorbate 80, found in many processed foods, might damage gut mucosa in mice, leading to leakage and inflammation.[34] Other researchers are studying the associations between dysbiosis and metabolic disease.[35] Michael Pollan reports on this in his interview with Patrice Cani, a biomedical scientist at the Universite Catholique de Louvain in Brussels. He writes: "When Cani fed a high fat, 'junk food' diet to mice, the community of microbes in their guts changed much as it does in humans on a fast-food diet. But Cani also found the junk-food diet made the animals' gut barriers notably more permeable, allowing endotoxins to leak into the bloodstream. This produced a low-grade inflammation that eventually led to metabolic syndrome." According to Pollan, Cani concluded that, "at least in mice, 'gut bacteria can initiate the inflammatory processes associated with obesity and insulin resistance' by increasing gut permeability."[36]

Finally, we know from new research that gluten (the consolidated proteins in wheat and related grains) can create problems in the gut. The story here is complex and related to both the findings about reduced mucus lining and the condition called "leaky gut," which we will discuss in chapter 8. For now, it is important to recall that different diets and environments are associated with differences in microbial composition, based on the studies of populations that inhabit or are exposed to the same food environments.[37] An individual's microbiome is often characterized as simultaneously stable for years regarding the species of certain microbes, but also very dynamic in the relative abundance of each species. Profiles of individuals' microbiomes vary widely, and we are only starting to understand how or why.

In sum, researchers have enabled us to know some of the pieces of the story connecting the microbiome to diet and health. We now know a fair amount about microbe health and its relation to the toxic things we eat. We know a little about foods and microbial communities in the gut, and we are learning more every day about the relationships between specific gut microbes and specific diseases and health, including the way that microbes not only aid digestion but also participate in processes necessary for health, for instance, the production of amino acids needed for the immune system. But at this point, we don't have studies of how modern foods that are drenched in pesticides (and that have questionable nutritional qualities) contribute to health or ill health by way of altering the microbiome. That is, there are no studies to date on how GM foods and pesticides might impact the microbiome in humans. Although some of the current research on the microbiome is largely agnostic when it comes to pesticides, there are a growing number of animal studies that show pesticides in food or absorbed through environmental exposure lead to diseases and immune disorders that are correlated with the microbiome.[38]

Food Is Information for the Microbiome . . . You Are What You Eat

Not all food is alike. This matters because food is a kind of information for the body's health; it provides the basic alphabet from which the prose of nutritional health is drawn. Let us explain the metaphor: Food contains a complex arrangement of nutrients that cannot be perfectly reproduced in vitamin pills or supplements alone. These nutrients include all the things that come together in whole, unprocessed food: phytochemicals, minerals, vitamins, and fiber, for instance. We are designed to process our food in ways that allow our genes to translate the environment into the vital substances of life. That is, the environment enters our bodies, and, once it is broken down into ingredients, the molecular bits of these ingredients, in effect, turn on or off genes, changing gene expression (although not changing the DNA itself), ultimately altering how our bodies function and determining its health. The microbiome plays a key role here.

Food arrives in the form of words, then, and it gets broken down, by digestion, into individual letters of the alphabet (molecules), *aided by the bacteria lining the gut*. Complex carbohydrates, like starches, need to be broken down into simple sugars in order to be assimilated into our bodies, but to do this we need the help of enzymes of specific bacteria. Once the word (the food) is broken down into its constituent letters (the molecules), some become a form of cellular instruction. We go from food to cellular instruction to genetic instruction—steps of biochemical transformation—creating proteins (chains of amino acids). These proteins are the building blocks of the body and thus are needed for everything—including healthy immune function, nerve function, nutrition of tissues, and so forth. This process of turning on and off genes to make certain proteins is what is meant by *epigenetics*. The changes are not to the genome (which comprises a sequence of nucleotides) but to the outside or 'epi' part of the gene, also known as DNA methylation and histone modification. These changes alter how genes are expressed—that is, "turning on and off" without changing the DNA sequence. It is important to remember that only certain food nutrients have the ability to affect gene function through epigenetic changes. This includes antioxidants such as EGCG (found in green tea), lycopene (found in tomatoes), and resveratrol (found in red grapes). The basic understanding is that only if our organs and tissues get this information will they function well. Digestion is affected, but so, too, are immunity, circulation, respiration, muscular response, and even cognition.

In addition to helping extract and store calories and nutrients from foods, however, microbes do more. Certain biota of the microbiome provide us with nutrients *that they themselves produce*.[39] For instance, *Bifidobacteria* can produce folate, a B vitamin that plays a crucial role in DNA synthesis and repair. When needed microbes are disrupted, or when they are absent, people get sick. These are the microprocesses that we worry about when it comes to eating foods that are compromised in their basic protein alphabet, or worse, in their transport of deleterious ingredients like pesticides.

There is a growing body of research on the impacts of pesticides on human health, but we are only starting to learn about the interplay of organic versus nonorganic foods, the microbiome, and epigenetic processes. At a minimum, however, it is safe to say that the environments in which foods are grown, and their health, likely both matter a great deal to human health, because foods are the most important informational sources for our biological system. Where foods come from and how they are grown determine the array of nutrients and quality of the foods themselves. A carrot is not created in a vacuum; it carries with it the history of how it was grown. Every food has a context, in other words, that is crucial to consider.

Perhaps the most important piece of the microbiome story is this: Whatever disrupts a healthy gut environment probably has significant impacts on the ways in which genes are turned off or on that, in turn, play a key role in regulating all of the body's physiology. This simple possibility serves as a beacon for researchers who are trying to connect the dots between the foods we put into our gut and health. Naturally occurring bacteria, but also antibiotics and pesticides such as glyphosate that has been patented as an antibiotic (explored more later), are things we now put into our guts in large quantities. Already, however, food-focused physicians and clinicians (including naturopaths, functional medicine doctors, and some non-Western medical practitioners) are linking these theories about food health and gut health and trying to relate them to what they are witnessing in their clinics. One proposition that links problems of a disrupted microbiome to chronic ailments is the disorder called leaky gut. Before we turn to leaky gut, however, we will return to Dr. Perro's clinic. Let's hear the story about Juan, who was exposed to, by both eating and absorbing, a *lot* of pesticides.

CHAPTER SEVEN

Unconventional Medicine for Treating Gut Dysfunction

The five Rs: remove, replace, reinoculate, repair, and rebalance.

THE CORE PRINCIPLES OF FUNCTIONAL MEDICINE

Gastrointestinal problems are one of most common reasons for pediatric visits.[1] Once acute etiologies like appendicitis are ruled out, clinicians must turn their attention to the biochemical, nutritional, and microbial possibilities. Still, few doctors use a diagnostic toolkit that enables them to decipher basic problems of the microbiome. We know the microbiome exists, but teaching students in medical schools how to test for a healthy microbiome is not yet standard (in part because the research is new) for anything except problems of chronic or recurring diarrhea and suspected IBS or colitis. But there are tests used by food-focused clinicians that look at gut dysfunction for a variety of other problems by looking through a different lens at the gut, and with these tests, a surprising number of abnormalities can be made visible.

Frequently the newest tests used by food-focused medicine are offered by biotechnology companies on the basis of the latest science, having been approved for use in humans but not yet fully incorporated into standard clinical practice guidelines. For a variety of reasons, clinical practice guidelines are often the last to change in response to biomedical research knowledge. Examples of these tests include polymerase chain reaction (PCR) tests for microorganisms in the gut, stool marker tests for inflammation, food immune response tests (IgG and IgA) for sensitivities and intolerances, tests for neurotransmitter levels in the urine (to assess neurobehavioral function), and tests for nutrient levels. We'll talk more about these in a moment. The clinical picture changes dramatically when you are using different tools to diagnose.

Food-focused clinicians who use these diagnostic tests are able to home in on problems with the gut, including inflammation, consequent immune system dysfunction, and a series of not just gastrointestinal issues but their sequelae in allergies, autoimmunity, and cognitive symptoms. These doctors have to go beyond laboratory work, as well. They are often taking diet inventories and working with sick children to figure out how to change their diets in ways that will heal their guts. Although integrative practices often veer off the conventional path, we need to pay attention to what these clinicians are saying and doing. These innovations are not risky in the sense that taking experimental new drugs can be; there are few to no risks when you're dealing with food, doing careful elimination diets. Some might argue that trying to solve problems this way might delay valuable conventional treatments that can reduce symptoms. But going along the conventional path can lead to dead ends and ongoing chronicity, a kind of Band-Aid treatment, as we've mentioned. We think it is useful to go in the other direction, to try a diagnosis and treatment protocol that might get to root problems by way of less palliative and more curative efforts that start with food. We need to pay attention to these integrative clinicians not only because they are getting results but also because patients and their families are driving the shift toward this form of care.

Juan's Descent into Dysbiosis and His Recovery with Food

Juan was a five-year-old boy who was brought in to Dr. Perro by his mom, Millie. Millie was emotionally worn down by the time she arrived at Dr. Perro's office, reporting that her son had been experiencing abdominal pain for the past six months. She described him as one minute being fine, playing with his brother. The next moment, he would be doubled over in pain. He reported "food burps" and a gassy tummy. His stool was either too hard or too runny, never normal. And he was having problems in kindergarten. Previously a happy-go-lucky guy, he was now persistently grouchy, oversensitive to touch, and had noticeably low energy. Millie described him as "not her son" when he acted like this.

Millie had brought Juan to his regular pediatrician. She said that he, too, was very concerned about Juan's tummy. He did routine blood work looking at Juan's cells that fight infection, took metabolic tests, screened for celiac disease, and did urine tests and stool cultures. That doctor reported that everything was "normal." Instead of validating Millie's suspicion that there was something physically causing Juan's problems, the doctor suggested that perhaps Juan was having a stress reaction from school or home and that she might want to consult a psychiatrist. In other words, Millie said, "He was trying to tell me that his symptoms were all 'in his head.'" This struck Millie as a diagnosis that was intended to dismiss her and her son's ailments rather than an actual prescription for further psychiatric care. It made her angry all the same. When she heard about Dr. Perro from a friend, she sought her out and made an appointment with her right away.

When Dr. Perro first met Juan, she noticed he had dark circles under his eyes, saw that he was pale, and detected a protruding abdomen and abnormally hyperactive bowel sounds. She ordered food antibody tests to see if he was having an immune response to any foods. She knew he didn't have any anaphylactic reactions—that is, he didn't have severe rashes, swollen tongue and throat, shortness of breath, vomiting, or changes in vital signs. There were no positive findings for IgE reactions, a true sign of allergy. Those events often occur during early exposures to certain foods, so a parent would likely know by this point in a child's life. But Dr. Perro tested for other antibodies (IgG and IgA). She also tested for nutrient levels such as zinc, magnesium, and vitamin B12 to understand if low levels of these nutrients were a contributing factor. Although the previous pediatrician did a thorough workup with the stool test and found nothing, Dr. Perro also ordered another stool analysis and culture, this time looking for markers of inflammation, infection, nutrient breakdown, and microbiome composition via genetic analysis (using PCR).

Using food sensitivity tests is a routine part of Dr. Perro's diagnostic repertoire. Most doctors don't use these tests because most food sensitivity reactions do not produce life-threatening situations, as true allergies do. There has also been controversy over the meaning of sensitivities and the ways in which they are tested. There are, in other words, different kinds of reactions the body can have to foods. The terminology is not entirely fixed, but a useful distinction might be that an *intolerance* comes from a lack of enzymes needed to digest that food (e.g., lactose intolerance). An *allergic* reaction stems from the body's mobilization of immune system histamines and IgE (immunoglobulin E), which can be life-threatening; whereas a *sensitivity* is a nonhistamine-producing immune reaction in which other antibodies are produced (e.g., IgA and IgG). Some scientists thought, and still think, that these IgA and IgG antibodies are a normal part of digestion. That is, all foods produce subtle immune reactions and this helps the body to digest. Dr. Perro and many others argue that these lesser antibody reactions are, in fact, a sign of a body in distress—and not a normal part of digestion.[2]

Clinically, these reactions often go away in kids who have been successfully treated—meaning they can return to eating those foods without producing antibodies. Dr. Perro also notes that children seem to have more immune reactivity than their parents to the same foods that the entire family consumes, suggesting dysfunction in the children's guts. This alone, she argues, suggests that normal digestion should not involve the immune system in this way. Juan was a good example.

Millie talked about how relieved she was that Dr. Perro was trying a different approach with Juan. Her commitment meant waiting for up to four weeks for some of the laboratory test results. But even before getting the results back, Dr. Perro decided it wouldn't hurt to get Juan onto a diet that would eliminate some of the common culprits that can cause gastrointestinal problems. First, she had him switch to a completely organic diet, something that would eliminate the amount of antibiotic and pesticide exposures he had. She also had him eliminate gluten and dairy from his diet, both of which are known to be a cause of inflammation in many kids. Eliminating them, she knew, would probably turn down the immune reaction and allow his gut to heal. Finally, she started him on supplemental probiotics and added homeopathic remedies designed for healing the gut.[3]

Initially, Millie was worried about making these changes to Juan's diet. She was concerned about the financial and also emotional costs of going completely organic, and she said that already they ate close to 50 percent organic anyway. She worried that the rest of her family would resist going off gluten and dairy, which would mean more work for her and having to prepare separate meals. Having never tried homeopathy or probiotics, even though she had heard of both, she was a little skeptical. Still, she went along with the plan.

Millie was shocked to see how much Juan improved in only *three* days after starting these dietary and supplemental treatments. She kept a log of his foods, and his symptoms, reporting that it was remarkable to see the change. By the time they came for their follow-up visit, she and Juan reported that his abdominal pain was lessened although still present, but the food burps were gone and his mood was hugely improved.

When Dr. Perro got the laboratory results back, she found much to report on. First, she found that Juan had very high immunoglobulin G (IgG) levels to both gluten and dairy, and he had IgG elevations to grains and citrus as well, although not to the same degree. He had low nutrient levels, which is known to affect mood, immune function, and mitochondrial function (responsible for energy production). His stool test showed that his microbial diversity was extremely low. His beneficial bacteria were almost nonexistent and he had overgrowth of several bacterial pathogens, including *Proteus mirabilis* and *Klebsiella pneumoniae*.

Dr. Perro turned to a mix of German Biological Medicines—Apo-Stom and Mundipur (remedies for extracellular matrix drainage) and SyGest (an immunomodulation remedy)—as well as herbs, supplemental vitamins and minerals, pre- and probiotics, and natural antimicrobials (such as oil of oregano) tailored to get rid of some of the unwanted pathogens, and to repair the gut. By his fourth visit, less than a year after they first met, Juan was back to his previous, happy self. The dark circles under his eyes were gone. His skin color was improved and his bowel findings were back to normal. His laboratory tests showed decreased immune markers, improved microbial diversity, and correction of nutrient deficiencies.

With cases like Juan's, one is always prompted to ask: What was the *real* culprit and what was the *real* source of his improvement? Was it the presence of unhealthy bacteria that were eradicated with natural antimicrobials? Was it the restoration of a normal balance of bacteria in the gut coupled with the removal of those that were unhealthy? Is it possible that his gut was already in a state of disrepair from other sources and that enabled harmful bacteria to settle in in the first place? Did his inflamed gut cause the sensitivities or were the foods he was eating creating the inflamed gut, causing a vicious cycle of dysfunctional digestion and damaged microbial environments? Was he experiencing psychological stress that added to his physical symptoms? Whatever the causes—and they were multiple, to be sure—we do know what worked to get him better.

Initially, with the simple removal of certain foods from his diet, his health was improved by the decrease in his chronic inflammation. Later, benefits came from tailoring his treatment so that some of the unwanted bacteria could be eradicated, and his dysbiosis reduced. What worked to get Juan healthy, in the end, was using a multipronged approach that restored a healthy balance of bacteria, eliminated unwanted bacteria, reduced inflammation by removing offending foods, and changed his diet to foods that would not damage his gut further. When his gut was repaired, his psychological and behavioral health improved as well. This approach is also known in functional medicine as the five Rs: remove, replace, reinoculate, repair, and rebalance.

Most people want singular, linear ways of explaining medical things. Linear models of cause and effect that explain singular named disorders are the normative models in conventional medicine. But the disorders we're talking about here that plague our kids these days are not so simple. They are usually multifactorial and have interrelated causal pathways. They are complex and point to a web of interrelated problems, often affecting multiple systems of the body at once. These problems tend to respond best not to singular interventions but to those that tie together multiple forms of therapy at once. In our review of clinical cases, a pattern stands out: Approaches that take food into account work far more often than they do not. Juan and many kids just like him get better and stay better by doing the many simple things clinicians like Dr. Perro prescribe. As Dr. Perro says, the complex problems we are witnessing today require a multimodal toolkit and an ability to try combinations of therapies in order to get our kids healthy.

By working with a theory of the relationship between foods and the gut, food-focused clinicians can connect the dots between chronic and persistent ailments and foods—connections that don't necessarily show up on the normal laboratory tests that doctors have in their diagnostic toolkits. It is important to remember that not only are the diagnostic tools sometimes divergent from what are used in conventional medicine but the theories of disease also diverge.

Dysbiosis, a general condition describing imbalance of the gut microbiome, is not a common diagnosis in pediatrician offices. And yet, dysbiosis is often at the heart of multiple ailments. Perhaps not surprisingly, there is no billing diagnostic code for it. In the next chapter, we will go into more detail about gut mechanics and offer another unconventional theory about gut dysfunction that will help explain how toxicants in our foods might be making our kids sick. Specifically, we will look at pathologic intestinal permeability, commonly known as "leaky gut."

CHAPTER EIGHT

Leaky Gut: A Key to Understanding Pesticide Impact on Health?

If our immune system is the body's Department of Defense, fighting off infection, gut microbes are the diplomats, determining what's harmful and what's harmless. The more robust the microbiota, the more sophisticated the diplomacy and the less likely the immune system will overreact and launch harmful autoimmune responses or fail to defend against invaders.

John Swansburg, from his article in *New York Magazine*, "Cute Family. And You Should See Their Bacteria"[1]

The characterization of the body as a system that works like the military, with combat zones and defense contractors, has prevailed for decades (think "fight the disease"). In this metaphor, the immune system is seen as having armies of cellular soldiers who go in pursuit of enemies, guarding our borders from invaders and keeping us protected with killer T cells and macrophages that gobble up the spoils of their battles.

In many ways, the combat metaphors are accurate. Anthropologist Emily Martin has written eloquently about how such metaphors came into being during our nation's most combat-driven eras, the years from World War I through the Vietnam War, when the engines of our political economy depended on the institutions of war and citizens were taught to identify with and embody their duty as soldiers.[2] These tactics served industrial capitalism well, Martin argues, disciplining citizens in ways that spilled over into our tactics for healing. She also reminds us that these metaphors were suited to a modern world in which fighting off infections and infectious pathogens was still the single most important task for health. But perhaps we have outgrown this way of relating to illness.[3]

Today, many of our most debilitating health problems are not a consequence of external pathogens that can be killed with better antibiotics. In fact, antibiotics have become one of our health hazards, and their overuse is a main cause in this generation's gut-related problems. Martin notes that not only have our models of immunity changed over time, but so, too, have the kinds of problems we now suffer from. Many of our morbidities today are consequences not of failing to keep enemies out, but rather a consequence of inner turmoil—that is, of autoimmune disorders in which the body attacks itself. Our bodies now fail because of their inability to distinguish between self and enemy, or where the body sees the self as the enemy.

What sorts of metaphors and what kinds of medicine are useful when the "enemy" has quite literally become our self? What would it mean to take seriously the notion that we should be focusing no longer on the body's combat units, T and B cells, but rather on its diplomats, the microbes, those skilled arbitrators who know that their own life and survival depend on their skillful negotiation for learning how to live with the enemy? Perhaps to live diplomatically by way of our gut means to live symbiotically, with an eye to how we might *both* survive (us and our microbial worlds). In the symbiotic world, what becomes important is striking a balance, a state of healthy equilibrium in which some microbes are nurtured and others are not, in which we recognize that living healthy means living with, and feeding, our microbial partners. This might be a particularly useful approach to dealing with problems of autoimmunity.

If we approached health from the insight that the microbiome is our first avenue for diplomacy—a form of negotiation between internal and external environments—what would medicine look like? How do we equip our microbiome to be good at diplomacy, to be skillful at helping us translate between the languages spoken both inside and outside of the body, attentive to the ways these translations are, in fact, key to health? Perhaps even the notion of diplomacy needs to be supplanted by a model of symbiosis—an approach that focuses on healthy cohabitation and sustainability, as described by scientist Lynn Margulis. Donna Haraway, who relies on Lynn Margulis's work, argues that this is a particularly feminist way of theorizing the world around us.[4] One might say that what has become important today under the scourge of autoimmune disorders is learning how to live *with others and ourselves* at the same time. We have to move past the model of combat and toward a model of symbiotic cohabitation. We must, as Haraway suggests, make kin with not just our microbes but with other surviving species cohabiting the ecosystem that we have put in peril.

Here is where research on the gut has become more exciting than ever, and where questions arise about what happens when we feed our microbiome toxicants. In the face of a constant barrage of toxicants—those chemicals we are literally bathing in—it is quite easy for the body to become overwhelmed, especially if it is not getting the nutrients it needs. Doctors sometimes refer to this as carrying too heavy an *allostatic* load—a situation in which homeostasis is compromised by multiple stressors. Chronic exposures to toxicants not only from our environment but also from our food result in a human-environmental imbalance, an allostatic situation where the whole ecosystem is overloaded.

If our bacteria play the most important role in our ability to navigate these challenges by being our first line of defense in detoxification, we must be sure they are cared for, fed, and nurtured. As Dr. Perro tells her patients, "Love your microbiome!" These microbes are our current biological diplomats—our navigators of symbiosis—but exactly what is their theater of combat is not so clear. Perhaps our current problems of autoimmune dysfunction are, in fact, telling us stories about the importance of the links between the environment and health, where we are our own greatest enemy.

One group of scientists who are helping us make sense of the relationships between the microbiome, food, and health are those working on "leaky gut" (otherwise known as intestinal permeability). Theories of leaky gut have been circulating in medicine for decades, but it has only been in the past decade or so that researchers have been able to put together a fine-tuned understanding of problems related to pathologies tied to intestinal permeability. Here, moving down to the microlevel of gut health, is where the current theater of combat is playing out, where self can become confused with enemy, and where the diplomatic skills of our microbes matter more than ever or, to move beyond the war metaphor, where we must learn to think of ourselves as symbiotic species cohabiting a mutual terrain that must be kept healthy. These microbes are representatives of and for our micro- and macroenvironment, our environmental ambassadors if you will, trying to help our internal worlds survive what we are doing to the world outside. What is going on in the microchambers of our guts where symbiosis can be disrupted, and what tools do we have for diagnosing and repairing these relationships?

Looking Deeper into Leaky Gut

Keep in mind that the gut—and specifically the small intestine—is designed to be a porous organ, not an impermeable boundary. It is designed to filter micronutrients (food that has been broken down into its constituent ingredients) from the digestive tract into the bloodstream and transport them to other organ systems, where they play a role in sustaining our structural integrity, tissue health, organ function, and physiological processes.

To understand leaky gut, we first need to revisit some basic facts about the intestines. The intestinal lining consists of one epithelial layer of cells that are folded into millions of fingerlike projections called villi, each of which is covered with cilia. Cilia help to transport micronutrients into the junctures that hold the epithelial cells together. In a healthy gut, these junctions remain fairly tight, enabling a fine-tuned screening of nutrients going into the blood, including amino acids, fats, key vitamins, and minerals that we have extracted from our foods. These nutrients can include wanted and unwanted by-products from microbes. They also can include toxicants.

A class of proteins that modulate the permeability of the epithelial junctures between cells is called *zonulin proteins*. Even though the gut is designed to be porous, scientists are now finding that the normal porosity of the gut can become impaired, inducing a greater number of openings that remain passable for a longer period of time, and therefore allowing larger products to enter the bloodstream. Having impaired gate functioning of the cells of the gut lining leads to the diagnosis of increased intestinal permeability, *leaky gut*.[5] With leaky gut, instead of having a tightly controlled, selective, and monitored lane of traffic, as if into a gated community, a wide, several-lane highway begins transporting substances from the digestive conduits into the blood.

Several things can go wrong to produce leaky gut. As we wrote about in chapter 6, if the bacteria that line the gut are starved by a lack of fiber, these bacteria will eat the mucus layer of the epithelium, creating raw sections of epithelium. These raw patches can impair intestinal function. Some argue that the development of raw sections of the gut, and its compromised mucosal protection, is a form of leaky gut. It is argued that this leaky gut, with its large swaths of exposed epithelium, promotes inflammation (that is, an immune response). Others argue for a more fine-tuned and somewhat different definition of leaky gut.

The current leading expert on leaky gut is a Harvard pediatrician and scientist named Alessio Fasano. His research discovered the mechanisms involved in celiac disease, a specific autoimmune disorder with a genetic predisposition in which the body, upon ingestion of gluten, attacks the lining of the small intestine. The genetics of celiac involve two HLA (human leukocyte antigen) markers.[6] Dr. Fasano figured out that people with celiac overproduce a molecule called *zonulin* in the presence of *gliadin*, one of the two molecular components of gluten (the other being *glutenin*). Zonulin, it turns out, is released when it comes into contact with gluten and, by bonding with it, creates holes in the lining of the intestinal wall, or the epithelium. Zonulin, in other words, is a gatekeeper for the lining of the epithelium. So when a person with a genetic predisposition to overproduce zonulin eats gluten, the villi of the intestinal lining become damaged with flattening of the villi, and more tight junctions are opened for sustained periods of time. This situation—a gut lining that is full of numerous holes that stay open for too long—is what physicians now call "increased intestinal permeability."

What Fasano's findings further show is that, over time, in the person predisposed to overproduce zonulin, more and more gluten proteins find their way into the bloodstream through these gaps in the intestinal lining. As a result, the body's immune system is stimulated, trying to eliminate these gluten proteins because they are seen as foreign. Over a long period of exposure, the immune system attacks the body's own villi.[7] Again, this condition is known as celiac disease. In 2000, Fasano reported that celiac occurred in roughly 1 out of 133 persons in the United States, although it appears that these numbers are increasing.[8]

Fasano's research shows that in addition to those with a genetic predisposition to overproduce zonulin (the celiac patient), there are at least two more common reactions to consumption of gluten. All people will have openings of the gut as a result of the ingestion of gluten, he says. In persons with a healthy immune system and no *overproduction* of zonulin, they will mount an immune response to the gluten particles that end up in the blood and clear them. This is a normal immune reaction to gluten. However, in people whose immune systems are compromised for one reason or another, there is chance of an extended inflammation reaction.

What Dr. Fasano is saying, as we understand it, is that even when people *without* the genetic predisposition to celiac disease eat gluten, there is a risk of epithelial disruption and immune response that can be problematic. In patients like this, there is the possibility of developing a *sensitivity* to gluten. People in this situation develop an immune response to gluten and, over time (with increased exposure to gluten), they too can develop autoimmune-like reactions. People with celiac and those with gluten sensitivities have high levels of zonulin in their blood. Fasano's work suggests, in other words, that some autoimmune diseases that have historically been associated with inheritance of parental DNA could, in fact, have additional causes. One of these is perhaps the DNA of organisms in the microbiome that can be altered by environment, exposure, and . . . you guessed it . . . foods.

Other researchers are studying gluten sensitivity. One group at Columbia University Medical Center offers the following explanation for the disorder, worth quoting at length:

> Researchers have struggled to determine why some people, who lack the characteristic blood, tissue, or genetic markers of celiac disease, experience celiac-like GI symptoms, as well as certain extra-intestinal symptoms, such as fatigue, cognitive difficulties, or mood disturbance, after ingesting foods that contain wheat, rye, or barley. One explanation for this condition, known as non-celiac gluten or wheat sensitivity (NCWS), is that exposure to the offending grains somehow triggers acute systemic immune activation, rather than a strictly localized intestinal immune response. Because there are no biomarkers for NCWS, accurate figures for its prevalence are not available, but it is estimated to affect about 1 percent of the population, or 3 million Americans, roughly the same prevalence as celiac disease. . . . [The participants with NCWS] did not have the intestinal cytotoxic T cells seen in celiac patients, but they did have a marker of intestinal cellular damage that correlated with serologic markers of acute systemic immune activation. The results suggest that the identified systemic immune activation in NCWS is linked to increased translocation of microbial and dietary components from the gut into circulation, in part due to intestinal cell damage and weakening of the intestinal barrier.[9]

What some researchers are now saying is that gluten sensitivity, which is more common than celiac disease, is likely associated with intestinal cell wall damage and increased gut permeability. In other words, the proposition is that preexisting dysbiosis can augment leaky gut and contribute to the development of gluten sensitivity. For patients who have a preexisting disorder, such as dysbiosis, gluten will not only augment the problem of gut leakiness, but also potentially augment the chances of developing sensitivity to gluten.

One can think up various scenarios. Imagine a child who has been on antibiotics frequently, or one whose microbiome was compromised early in life (by being born via Caesarean section, for instance). This child may develop problems from eating gluten, perhaps from increased zonulin (holding the junctions open) or perhaps from inflammation resulting from fiber-deprived or dysbiotic patches in the lining of the gut (from other causes). This all makes the gut even leakier, simultaneously triggering immune responses and possibly a state of chronic immune system activation. While all this is happening, the gut is not doing its job effectively, failing to break down food adequately and pass needed nutrients into the bloodstream, but also allowing large unwanted particles to get into the bloodstream. It is a vicious cycle of digestive malfunction. Add to this the possibility of toxicants getting into the bloodstream by this route, and you get . . . a very sick kid.

Why Are Autoimmune Disorders on the Rise?

There is not a lot of definitive knowledge about the etiological mechanisms of autoimmunity, although there are theories. Inflammatory bowel diseases, such as ulcerative colitis and Crohn's disease, are gastrointestinal autoimmune diseases that are on the rise in our kids. What concerns us is that if we accept that gluten sensitivity and abnormal intestinal permeability exist in many individuals, and that low-grade leaky gut has been around for many years, why are we seeing increasing rates of chronic abdominal disorders (including leaky gut) in children *now*? What are the links between the rise in gluten sensitivity, the rise in autoimmunity, and the rise of so many other digestive symptoms?

We believe dysbiosis explains a lot and points us in the direction we need to go to understand autoimmunity. Consider these connections: We rely on microbes for the production of aromatic amino acids such as *tyrosine*, *phenylalanine*, and *tryptophan*. One of their functions is that they are the precursors of the production of chemicals that transmit neurologic signals (neurotransmitters), but they are also widely utilized in many of the body's functions. When the organisms that assist in their production are suboptimal or imbalanced (including *E. coli* and *Corynebacterium glutamicum*), we see disruptions in biological systems. Thyroid function, sleep, hormonal and neurotransmitter production, as well as the immune system, all become compromised. The healthy microbiome is also a key producer of vitamin B12, thiamine, riboflavin, and vitamin K.[10] When the gut is leaky or impaired (dysbiotic), not only is the body *not* getting proper nutrition from its food, it is also not getting proper nutrition from its microbiome, because the microbiome is itself not getting its own proper nutrition. What happens when this vicious cycle gets set in motion?

One of the things that can go wrong in the gut when it is dysbiotic is that bacteria that normally reside in the colon can migrate up to the small intestine. As harmful bacteria are allowed to populate the small intestine, they also release toxins such as *lipopolysaccharides*, signaling activation of the immune system.[11] These migrations can also increase the production of zonulin, further exacerbating the gut's leakiness and producing symptoms such as diarrhea. A leaky gut does not efficiently absorb food nutrients, and it allows large unwanted particles to enter the bloodstream or to pass through the digestive tract incompletely digested. Abnormal particles in the bloodstream can trigger low-grade immune system activation because they are seen as foreign invaders. Could chronic leaky gut produce a chronic overstimulation of immune reactions and, because of compromised nutrition, could the immune system be overreactive but undereffective? Like a faulty car engine, does it muster a persistent effort of growls and sputters, but can it not ultimately start up? Is this in part what is going on with autoimmunity? Is dysbiosis (leading to leaky gut) a root cause of many of our kids' chronic autoimmune disorders?

So, to return to the question of why the rise in gluten sensitivity, chronic autoimmune problems, and the epidemic of gastrointestinal disorders, we wonder if there are other causes of leaky gut than just gluten and known pathogenic bacteria? Could things like toxicants and antibiotics (or *pesticides that are antibiotics*) be getting into the gut to produce or augment leakiness or trigger chronic immune reactions? We think so. Are chronic disorders a result of chronic exposures to toxic chemicals that are destroying our children's guts?

We could also talk about functional disorders that manifest in different systems of the body far from the digestive tract. These include endocrine disorders (e.g., diabetes), atopic disorders (e.g., asthma, eczema, and allergy), and also cognitive problems (e.g., autism spectrum disorder, ADHD, developmental delays, and a variety of other mood disorders).

Could dysbiosis and leaky gut play some role in all of these problems as connectors that link microbiome problems with chronic diseases?

The model of disorders we are talking about in this book recognizes that many systems are involved, that they are interactive, and that they create situations of mutual exacerbation that result in symptoms that we don't fully understand. All of these possible routes to sickness are potentially present in adults, and they beg the question about food as a source of not only nourishment and health, but also pathogenesis. What happens when our foods themselves contain chemicals that are known to be harmful to us or to our microbiome? What happens when these chemicals pass through leaky membranes of the gut into the bloodstream? Because children, and especially infants, are still developing a healthy microbiome and immune system, they might be particularly vulnerable to even small exposures to things that disrupt normal function of the gut. Let's look at another family who had to confront these issues directly.

Celiac Disease and Sensitivity in the Family

Caroline came to see Dr. Perro because both of her sons were sick, and so was she. She had recently, at age forty, been diagnosed with celiac disease, having experienced disabling abdominal pain, bloating, diarrhea, reflux, and rashes for most of her life. Caroline reported that both her sons, ages ten and twelve, also had chronic abdominal pain. She asked Dr. Perro to evaluate them for celiac disease as well.

Quentin, Caroline's ten-year-old son, had a history of chronic abdominal pain and fit the description of having "failure to thrive" (not gaining adequate weight or height over a prolonged period of time). Dr. Perro learned that Quentin had IgG antibodies to gluten, as well as to other foods, and that he possessed both HLA genetic markers associated with celiac disease. Often, kids with celiac are offered an intestinal biopsy to confirm the diagnosis of celiac, but Caroline did not want to put her son through this invasive procedure. Because of Caroline's diagnosis and because Quentin had two of the HLA genetic markers along with significant IgG antibodies to gluten, Dr. Perro recommended an all-organic diet, removal of gluten, a regimen of homeopathics, and probiotic supplements to heal his intestinal lining. Within several months, Quentin not only got rid of his abdominal pain, but he also began to grow.

Quentin's twelve-year-old brother, Stephan, was thriving in comparison to Quentin, even though he also was having chronic abdominal pain. Stephan also had significant IgG markers for gluten and other foods, but tested positive for only one celiac gene, the less common variant. (Having these genes does not necessarily mean that you will develop celiac disease, but anyone with celiac disease has one or the other of these markers.) Dr. Perro guessed that Stephan was gluten sensitive but not celiac at the time she treated him. When Caroline eliminated gluten from his diet as well, Stephan's symptoms resolved. In fact, all three family members were helped immensely by a therapy that not only removed gluten from their diets, but that also focused on efforts to heal the gut and restore a healthy microbiome in part by switching to organic.

Dr. Perro sees hundreds of patients like this family, year in and year out: patients who come to see her who have had lifelong problems with their digestion but who remain without a diagnosis. Conventional treatment for kids with celiac is well established: Remove the gluten from the diet. But for those who don't have a diagnosis of celiac, who still suffer from digestive problems, there are few recommendations and few diagnoses. Dr. Perro's approach was to treat both kids as if they were unable to tolerate gluten and to assume they had leaky guts. Treatment was focused on getting their guts healthy. As with other patients, she also guessed that getting rid of pesticides by switching to organic foods would help.

Cases like that of Caroline and her two sons demonstrate diversity within families. There are kids with celiac genes with symptoms of the disease, kids with celiac genes without symptoms of full-blown celiac, and kids with symptoms that resemble celiac disease but who don't have the genetic markers. In other words, sensitivity to gluten can be related to problems other than celiac, perhaps even arising in kids with guts that are leaky for reasons that have nothing to do with gluten. What we don't know yet is *why this is the case*. We think it has to do with chronic exposure to toxicants.

In diagnosing health by way of the gut, we turn our attention to what we are feeding our microbiome. This includes paying attention to foods that we might or might not be able to digest, but it also includes looking at the possibility of toxic substances inside of our foods that might be harming the gut. What is the evidence that this is happening, that the foods we are eating are gut harmful? One way to answer this question is to explore our food production systems. Are the things we do to grow our food making our food dangerous? In order to answer this, we first want to back up and look at what happens when our kids are exposed to the same inputs that our industrial food system is exposed to. That is, what happens when kids are exposed to pesticides? Let's take another look at the clinical manifestations of leaky gut arising from chronic exposure to pesticides. We'll now turn to the story of Zoe, whose exposure to pesticides sprayed near her home made her very sick.

CHAPTER NINE

Chronic Exposure: Contamination as a Way of Life

Ironically, the more knowledgeable we are about a problem, the more we are filled with a paralyzing futility. Futility, in turn, forestalls action. But action is exactly what is necessary to overcome futility.

SANDRA STEINGRABER,
author of *Raising Elijah*[1]

A theory of intestinal permeability in relation to the microbiome cannot explain everything, but it goes a long way toward a deeper understanding of chronic illness. In fact, we believe leaky gut and dysbiosis potentially explain a lot of old problems—problems that have always existed even though we didn't have explanations for them, and that are now on the rise. We argue, in fact, that these problems are reaching epidemic levels, and so we should be looking at their causes in new ways.

In this book we have explored some of the possible reasons for microbiome disruption and intestinal permeability. In chapter 4, we explored other toxicants that are impacting our children's health: toxic chemicals that penetrate the body through the lungs, the skin, and the mouth that can have direct negative effects on the body. We saw how environmental health scholars and researchers are bravely mapping the presence and harms of contaminants that many of our children are exposed to on a daily basis. They tell us that chemical pollutants that come from factories, automobile exhaust, and metals in our drinking water are all around us, but they are also in drywall, PVC pipes, plastic food packaging, toys, water bottles, paper receipts, cosmetics, detergents, flame retardants, and dry-cleaning products, to name only a few. But we are also exposed to toxic chemicals from our foods and our food production systems. Contamination from chemical pollutants has become an unavoidable and normal way of life.

Scholars of environmental science and toxicology alert us to our false sense of security in relation to chemicals. Their insights are useful for understanding how we have gone wrong with foods. For example, because we wash our hands in soap, therefore eliminating infection from microorganisms, we feel we are "safe" from contamination. Indeed, we conceptualize surfaces as "clean" if they are free from dirt and bacteria. But this is just wrong. Most cleaning products, plastic goods, and processes we use to ensure cleanliness leave invisible and harmful chemical residues. The notion of "a clean countertop fit to eat off of" is anything but safe. In fact, some microbiome researchers and writers have proposed the opposite is true. Not only are chemicals in many of our cleaning products neurotoxic and carcinogenic, but many of the bacteria they kill are actually vital to development of a healthy microbiome. Scholars now say that to stay healthy we must train our microbiome and immune system early on by frequently exposing ourselves to bacterial pathogens, not creating an environment where they don't exist. This is called the *hygiene hypothesis*, and is explored by microbiologists like B. Brett Finlay (whose work we discussed earlier in chapter 6).

We know that a robust microbiome that helps to produce healthy immune responses is the opposite of a leaky dysbiotic gut. Researchers, like Martin Blaser (whom we also learned about in chapter 6) and Moises Velasquez-Manoff (author of *An Epidemic of Absence*) write that ingestion of some microbes might be the essential safeguard against autoimmune diseases, such as Crohn's disease and multiple sclerosis.[2] Researchers have argued that children who grow up in close contact with farm animals, such as Amish children, tend to have lower rates of childhood asthma compared to other communities.[3]

The fact that we are killing off useful bacteria in our environment is as bad as the fact that we are using chemicals that are known to produce health problems. These problems are related. When we live in a toxic environment, we are putting our own internal biological flora and fauna at risk. So, even if we have avoided the problem of oversanitization, we could still be putting our kids at risk by unknowingly exposing them to toxic chemicals that harm these useful gut bacteria. What happens when children are chronically exposed to toxicants? They get sick.

Clinicians trying to treat children they suspect are being exposed to environmental toxicants often face a dilemma. There is a significant difference between the evaluation of a child with an acute poisoning (a child accidentally sprayed by pesticides or a toddler who drank an unmarked bottle of a pesticide, for example) and a child who has long-term, ongoing exposure to the same pesticides. There are toxicologic decontamination guidelines for acute poisonings, and entire departments in hospitals and in county clinics are set up to manage these types of problems. However, there is sparse information available to the clinician for diagnosis, testing, and treatment of children who have been subjected to long-term, daily, nonlethal, lower-dose exposures.

Zoe: A Case of Toxic Exposure

Take the case of Zoe, a six-year-old child from a wine-growing region of California, who was brought to Dr. Perro when she was three years old. Zoe's mom, Debbie, reported that she was "going out of her mind" caring for Zoe. She now had a new infant and didn't have the patience to deal with Zoe's constantly swinging moods and outbursts. She described living with Zoe as like living with Dr. Jekyll and Mr. Hyde.

Zoe would tantrum uncontrollably when other children were sitting patiently at circle time in preschool. She had aggressive outbursts of biting and hitting other children, often unprovoked. She had a difficult time falling asleep, but still often woke up at 4:30 in the morning, raring to go. Debbie found herself constantly frazzled and distraught. She spoke to her regular pediatrician and was referred to a child psychiatrist. The psychiatrist recommended that Zoe take Risperdal, a medication used for patients with psychosis. Debbie went online and read about this drug. What she found made her feel desperate and horrified because it was a drug for serious cases of psychosis with many side effects. She didn't think Zoe was psychotic, and the side effects seemed possibly worse than the symptoms. Zoe's behavior seemed far beyond what one might expect from an older sibling after the arrival of a new baby into the home. Debbie felt that the issue was biological, not psychological, but she was not keen on using this drug. However, she was afraid to do nothing. She was fearful that Zoe would be thrown out of yet another preschool, and this was a hardship she couldn't bear, as both she and her husband needed to work full time. When Debbie talked to her friend and neighbor about it, her neighbor mentioned that her own child had been having behavioral issues but had been successfully treated by Dr. Perro without use of strong antipsychotic medications. So, Debbie made an appointment with Dr. Perro.

Dr. Perro did a patient intake that lasted an hour and a half (her normal time frame for the long history taken on a first visit). Even though Zoe was brought in for behavioral issues, she clearly had a lot of digestive and gut problems. She regularly had severe constipation and abdominal bloating. Dr. Perro listened to Debbie as she listed her numerous concerns about Zoe's behavior. When Dr. Perro learned that they lived near an agricultural area, on the edge of many vineyards, she started to consider the impact from Zoe's likely exposure to pesticides. She also found out from Debbie that there were other neighbors who had kids struggling with behavioral problems. She suspected environmental toxicants might be at work based on all these things: the behavioral, clearly neuropsychological issues; the fact that Zoe lived where she did; and the added symptom of her constipation, which Dr. Perro suspected meant she wasn't properly eliminating her toxicant-laden waste.

Dr. Perro then suggested that the families in Debbie's neighborhood collaborate and do a soil analysis. What they found shocked them. It turns out they were all living across the street from a leach field that was filled with toxic chemicals. The pieces of the puzzle were coming together.

To figure out how to go forward from there, Dr. Perro ran a urinary environmental pollutants profile on Zoe. The results were, again, shocking. Zoe showed extreme elevations of all chemical groups that were tested for—petrochemicals, styrenes, plastics, and parabens—demonstrating that she was being exposed to significant amounts of chemicals. Some of these chemicals are known neurotoxins, as well as carcinogenic. They were at much higher levels than in the average child, upward of the 95th percentile in terms of her levels of contamination. Essentially, she was off the charts.

The first approach to treating Zoe involved trying to diminish her exposure to the chemicals by eliminating the offending agents. *Remove.* This meant helping the family to detoxify their home. Later Dr. Perro would help Debbie figure out ways to get the school and neighborhood involved in trying to clean up the school and the leach field. Both of these last efforts were unsuccessful. The school was resistant to the idea that pesticides were in any way involved in causing harm to their students. The county refused to do any type of toxic cleanup on the lot because it was not identified as a Superfund site. There simply weren't funds, but they also didn't want to acknowledge any tie between the children's health and the field.

Focusing on the patient in front of her, Dr. Perro turned to the work of toxicologists and tried to find ways to help Zoe's body to eliminate the chemicals. For instance, she prescribed an amino acid protocol along with antioxidants and certain B vitamins that would improve cellular processes needed for detoxification—helping the liver to clear toxicants. In order to see how well Zoe was able to methylate, one means by which the liver is able to detoxify chemicals from the body, Dr. Perro ran a genetic profile, specifically looking at her methylation genetics—the MTHFR (methyltetrahydrofolate reductase enzyme) status test. She learned that Zoe was homozygous for one of the genes she needed to properly methylate—she had a defective MTHFR gene. This went a long way toward explaining why Zoe, but not all the other kids in her neighborhood, was affected so severely by the toxicants she was exposed to. She needed a supplement that would enable this methylation to happen (methyl B12, glutathione, and N-acetyl cysteine, or NAC). *Replace.* It also affirmed the possibility that her behavioral problems were largely a result of this combination of the defective methylation gene and, consequently, the presence of toxicants in her body and brain.

In addition to getting Zoe's mom to put her on an all-organic diet, and taking her off gluten and dairy until she could do more specific tests for sensitivities to foods, Dr. Perro also prescribed probiotics from the first visit. Regarding the strong links between the healthy gut and the healthy brain, described in chapter 6, the goal here was to improve cognitive and behavioral function by way of reintroducing specific healthy and beneficial microbes to her gut. *Reinoculate.* Healing often comes in stages, but getting the gut healthy is usually the first step. Dr. Perro knew that no matter how effective her protocols to improve detoxification were, without a healthy gut (even to digest the supplements) there would be little progress. She treated with specific strains and high colony counts of *Lactobacilli* and *Bifidobacteria*. But to help Zoe's brain, she treated with essential fatty acids, including combinations of omega three and omega six fatty acids. *Repair.*

Over several months, Zoe made slow and steady improvement. Her mood swings diminished and she was much more stable emotionally. Her aggression resolved. Her sleep improved. Her constipation resolved. Dr. Perro also layered in other types of therapies, including osteopathic manipulative medicine (to rebalance the musculoskeletal system) as well as cognitive behavioral therapy (a form of psychotherapy). *Rebalance.* Although Debbie had tried the latter before and found it unhelpful, they were now able to implement this therapy with great success. With the strong links between the gut and the brain, it makes sense that psychotherapies and the manipulative work were only effective *after* Zoe's gut was healed.

Zoe's case offers a good example of how behavioral problems can be ameliorated by diagnostic tools that consider chronic exposure to toxicants as a possible source of pathogenesis. It also illustrates how healing efforts work best when tackled through a multipronged approach, which might include figuring out the genetic profile of the child and correcting for that, examining the condition of the gut and repairing it, and using direct efforts to eliminate exposure to offending toxicants.

The Dangers of Well-Informed Futility

Sandra Steingraber, a leading science writer on the dangers of environmental toxicants to children's' health, uses the psychologist Gerhardt Weibe's notion of *well-informed futility* to describe how even people who understand the risks they face will do nothing about it. In Weibe's case, it was the problem of televised overinformation that gave rise to a sense of futility over warfare; in Steingraber's it was the problem of how people who *knew* the risks their children faced from environmental toxins still wouldn't do anything to change it. She calls it a form of *learned helplessness*.[4] This is what we initially witnessed with Zoe's case when her school and county would not help.

We are faced with the same issue when it comes to environmental toxicity. The problem is that the task of fixing the environment feels utterly overwhelming, and there is too great a temporal distance between exposures and the development of chronic and sometimes deadly disorders. The truth is, the task *is* overwhelming. Individuals cannot do much to change the infrastructural conditions of the built environment around them without investing significant time and money, just as they cannot single-handedly change the quality of the air they breathe. These things have to be done in the realm of policy and policy enforcement. Even there, though, things get slippery.

If we start from an environmental health sciences perspective, it is easy to see how, often, the things we do to protect and improve our lives end up harming us. Just as our cleaning products and efforts to eradicate microbial pathogens to make us healthier turn out to sometimes have the opposite effect, our modern food production systems have also produced unintended harmful consequences that were deployed, initially, in the name of food safety. A clear picture of how these technologies are causing health problems is needed before any change can be made in this regard, both at an individual and at a societal level. But, even here, developing a clear picture of this science is not easy.

One need only spend a short amount of time looking into the science behind modern food to learn that controversy over the actual risks of pesticide exposure relies on information that is highly contested. This includes information in sensational media coverage and diatribes by internet bloggers as well as actual scientific studies funded by organizations on both sides of the fence. Information in peer-reviewed articles that are written by scientists and are available in science archives of PubMed is perhaps the hardest to decipher when it comes to the facts about health risks of pesticides, for example. This is not a case of *learned helplessness*, as Steingraber described, as much as it is a problem of obfuscation and lack of reliable information, along with a huge amount of contestation over the facts. Despite the existence of a lot of information on modern food, there is a lack of clarity, as competing claims about how these foods might or might not impact health vie for attention and monopolies on the truth.

Perhaps the single most contested, obfuscated, and unreliable issue of modern industrial food production is the use of GM technologies. As we mentioned in chapter 4, the argument put forward by agribusiness industries and many food scientists is that GM food technologies were designed to help us and continue to help us *reduce* the amount of toxic chemicals needed in conventional agriculture. GM technologies in foods, we are told, were created as biological, as opposed to chemical, techniques to control pests and weeds in ways that were safe for humans. These techniques were designed to reduce the burden on the agricultural industry and make it possible to "feed the world" with commodity foods. But what if the very effort to make our foods safer and more plentiful has actually resulted in a situation in which our foods are more toxic than ever, our environment more polluted than ever, and our food supply at more risk than ever in the history of modern industrial agriculture? Over the next three chapters we will explore all these issues. First, in chapter 10, we will look at what genetically modified foods are, exploring the chemicals they were designed to be used with, along with a deep dive into the regulatory blind spots about them. In chapter 11, we will explore the growing body of evidence in support of, and the counterevidence against, the safety of GM foods. Finally, in chapter 12, we'll look specifically at the case of the most commonly used pesticide in relation to GM foods, Roundup, and its active ingredient, glyphosate.

CHAPTER TEN

The Making of Modern Industrialized Food

Back then, industrial agriculture was hailed as a technological triumph that would enable a skyrocketing world population to feed itself. Today, a growing chorus of agricultural experts—including farmers as well as scientists and policymakers—sees industrial agriculture as a dead end, a mistaken application to living systems of approaches better suited for making jet fighters and refrigerators.

UNION OF CONCERNED SCIENTISTS,
United States[1]

What we call "modern" food is food that has been grown using intensive agrochemical industrial methods. It is mass-produced, high-technology, and chemical-dependent food. It is monocrop and livestock sources of food. It is not organic food. It is not locally produced organic food. It is the kind of food that has led to massive subsidies for corn, soybean, and wheat farmers across the United States, and that now relies on massive supplies of chemical fertilizers and pesticides. The key aspect of industrial foods that we are interested in and, in part, that fostered these chemical dependencies is, as mentioned, GM crops.

Although genetic-modification techniques were developed in the late 1970s and early 1980s (in tobacco plants), GM foods only entered the food supply in the United States in 1994 with the Flavr Savr tomato (a tomato genetically engineered to have a long shelf life).[2] The first GM-food row crop (soybeans) was introduced in 1996. Since that time, the use of GM technologies has grown fast and far with foods produced in the United States. In 2016, 94 percent of all soybeans grown in the United States were genetically modified, as were 92 percent of all corn, 93 percent of cotton, and 95 percent of sugar beets, and in 2006, 87 percent of the canola grown in the United States (and 90 percent of canola grown in Canada) was genetically modified, though these numbers change slightly every year.[3] Papaya, zucchini, and summer squash are also available with genetic modifications, with nearly 90 percent of the papayas grown in Hawaii modified to protect against the ringspot virus. (Hawaii is actually where a huge amount of the experimentation to develop GM crops takes place.[4]) The GM Arctic apple has just been launched, and, historically, GM technologies have been used in strawberries as well. GM potatoes have also recently been relaunched with a variety known as Innate, engineered not to brown so easily when cut. There are different traits that are engineered for specific crops: some that make the plants insect-killers, some that enable them to resist herbicides, and some that enhance specific qualities (such as the amount of vitamin A they have, or their resistance to frost). Often GM traits are "stacked," meaning multiple modifications can be made to one plant.

Genetic modification is also used in production of legumes (including alfalfa used in feed for livestock) and dairy products. A GM hormone (rBGH or rBST) is also frequently injected into some dairy cows in the United States to make them produce more milk, although farmer uptake has markedly reduced in the past years.[5] Canada and Europe have banned use of this hormone. Finally, GM technologies are used in food additives, such as aspartame, enzymes, added flavorings, and processing agents, as well as in yeasts used to make wine.[6] What is important to note here is that GM foods and animals that eat GM foods (or have been injected with GM hormones) have been around in our commercial food system for only the past few decades, decades in which our current generation of children and teens have been consuming them.

The invention and dissemination of GM technologies in our foods have spawned a huge controversy in which scientists have become divided, along with the public. Questioning the safety of these foods and, conversely, insisting on their safety form two poles of the debate. In the next few chapters, we will explore this debate, including the ways in which it forms a politics of knowledge that often obscures truths as often as it reveals them. We will learn more about who is involved with the debate as well as the factual claims that people on both sides are making in the next chapter.

Here, at the outset, we want to clarify that we are not trying to convince readers that all genetic modification is wrong. In fact, a good deal of benefit has and will continue to come from using GM and transgenic technologies, particularly in the field of medicine. Gene therapies are potentially useful to eliminating genetic diseases from embryos (although this is very controversial) and already GM technologies are used to make insulin and other drugs. There are potentially many beneficial uses of GM technologies for genetically inherited health problems. These technologies are, however, rigorously tested on human subjects before they are rolled out for general use. As we have seen, this is not the case for GM foods.

There are very important reasons to be concerned about GM foods. We know that GM technologies *have changed* the composition of many of the foods we eat, by definition. GM technologies do not just enhance or change foods the way that natural hybridization techniques do, as we will see. While agrochemical industries nevertheless say these foods are nutritionally *equivalent* to non-GM foods (and on this basis are not subjected to further study before being sold to the public), there is a growing body of evidence that this is not the case.

The most widely debated and controversial of the GM foods are those we began to talk about in chapter 4: Roundup Ready and Bt toxin crops. These two crops constitute over 99 percent of all commercialized GM crops grown at present.[7] The commercialized Roundup Ready crops include soy, corn, canola, alfalfa, cotton, sugar beets, and potatoes and, possibly soon, wheat.[8] A small handful of companies own patents on Roundup Ready seeds. Farmers today must purchase Roundup Ready seeds every year if they want to use Roundup (and other glyphosate-based herbicides). In the past, farmers were usually able to reuse seed from one year's crop to the next. This practice is not allowed with GM crops. Farmers must repurchase their seeds every year for every crop.

Bt, or *Bacillus thuringiensis*, crops are crops that have been genetically engineered so that the toxic capacities of the Bt are expressed as a genetic trait of the plant itself. As we explained, the plant becomes an insecticide that can kill various pests, such as the European corn borer, southwestern corn borer, tobacco budworm, cotton bollworm, pink bollworm, and Colorado potato beetle. We'll talk more about Bt crops and their mechanisms later. Here, it is useful to know that there is agreement among those both for and against GM foods about the basic biochemical mechanisms of these crops and the ubiquity of them in our food. Beyond that, things get controversial very quickly. So, how do they work?

Glyphosate and Roundup Ready Foods

Roundup Ready or glyphosate-tolerant crops are genetically modified to withstand the spraying of glyphosate-based herbicides, the best known of which is Monsanto's Roundup. That is, Roundup Ready plants are not killed by the herbicide Roundup, or more specifically by its primary active ingredient, glyphosate. In other words, Roundup can be used indiscriminately to kill weeds without killing the crop plants as well.

Glyphosate was first patented in 1964 by the Stauffer Chemical Company as a metal chelator, used to clean metal pipes. Coincidentally, it was observed that the plants in the areas where it was being used had been killed, prompting research on its use as an herbicide. It was subsequently patented as an herbicide ingredient by Monsanto, which began to sell it to farmers in 1974. From 1974 to 1991, Monsanto became the market leader in the production of glyphosate-based broad-spectrum herbicide. After its patent expired in 1991, the company retained a patent on the isopropyl amine salt, which is the most widely used salt form for glyphosate, thereby retaining its patent protection in the United States until 2000. Today, many companies make glyphosate-based products, though Monsanto maintains its market share by packaging its GM Roundup Ready seeds together with its own brand of glyphosate-based herbicide, Roundup.

When sprayed on a weed, glyphosate is absorbed, with the aid of a mixture of poorly disclosed adjuvants (often misleadingly labeled "inert" or simply "other") in the commercial formulation, through the plant's foliage and roots. Once inside the plant, it inhibits an enzyme (EPSPS) involved in the synthesis of three amino acids: tyrosine, tryptophan, and phenylalanine. Glyphosate works to kill a weed by interrupting what is called the *shikimate* pathway. The shikimate pathway is a seven-step metabolic route used by bacteria, fungi, algae, parasites, and plants for the biosynthesis of aromatic amino acids (phenylalanine, tyrosine, and tryptophan). In the absence of these aromatic amino acids, the weed's synthesis of proteins is blocked and so it dies.

The makers of Roundup have argued that since human and animal cells do not have the shikimate pathway, it is safe for them. In fact, when it was invented it was marketed as a promising herbicide precisely because it was thought to have no effect on humans and animals. We now know, however, that the bacteria in our microbiome *do* have the shikimate pathway. We also know that in vitro studies (laboratory studies performed in flasks or dishes) suggest that when glyphosate-saturated foods are eaten, the microbiome might be saturated in glyphosate as well, which we'll discuss in chapter 11. This is not surprising considering that Monsanto also applied for a patent on glyphosate *as an antibiotic* in 2002 and was granted the patent by the US patent office in 2010.[9]

Monsanto started selling commercial Roundup Ready seeds in 1996, pitching the benefits to farmers for controlling weeds without killing their crop plants. For farmers, it was hard to resist. Another supposed benefit to using Roundup Ready seeds was that they also offered a short-term reduction in the amount of fertilizer needed in growing the crop (since the weeds were decimated by use of Roundup, less fertilizer was needed to help the crop compete with weeds). Over time, however, these genetically engineered crops have spurred the growth of more and more Roundup-resistant weeds (from selection pressure, whereby only those weeds that resist the herbicide survive to proliferate). Farmers who had been using glyphosate-based herbicides year after year were beginning to find that their weeds had adapted, and sprang up regardless of how much Roundup they used on their crops. As a result, farmers have had to use mixtures of herbicides and higher rates of glyphosate herbicide, as weed resistances steadily increase. Thus the idea that Roundup-resistant seeds would require less pesticide use was short-lived, along with the idea that these technologies would ensure higher yields, a point we will revisit later.[10] Critics argue that pesticide use has exponentially increased over time, and this is a boon to industry.

In addition to the escalation in use of glyphosate on Roundup Ready crops, glyphosate is also apparently being used as a desiccant or ripening/drying agent on *non*-Roundup Ready crops, protecting them from moisture-related loss. That is, crops such as edible peas and small grains such as oats, wheat, and barley are apparently sometimes being sprayed in some places as soon as three to eight days pre-harvest with glyphosate-based herbicides to prevent sprouting. This action, which might reduce unwanted variables for the agricultural industry at the time of harvest, puts residue of a powerful chelator and potent antibiotic *directly* into the food supply. Our concern is that this increase in glyphosate in the food supply correlates with the rise of chronic immune and digestive disorders/dysbiosis.

Bt Toxin GM Crops

The second kind of GM crop that concerns us is the input of naturally occurring toxins into a plant's DNA. This technology enables companies to turn plants themselves into insecticides. These plants are registered as pesticides with the EPA. There are many different versions of this GM technique, but we will focus on Bt toxin (*Bacillus thuringiensis*).

Bt is a naturally occurring soil-dwelling bacterium. The protein toxin derived from it has been used for decades by farmers, including organic farmers, to get rid of unwanted pests from plant crops. The way it works is like this: The insect eats the Bt toxin protein. The Bt toxin dissolves in the high pH insect gut and becomes active, releasing a crystal, or Cry, protein. The activated Bt toxin then inserts into the gut wall of the insect, essentially punching holes in the lining of the gut. These holes allow bacteria in the insect gut to enter its body, where they multiply. The insect dies of a type of septicemia.[11]

Again, farmers have for many years sprayed (and some still do) Bt toxin onto their crops to kill pests. Applied as a spray, the Bt toxin breaks down and dissipates with exposure to sun and moisture. It can be reapplied over time if pests return. But, applied in this way, this pesticide can be largely eliminated from the plant before it is consumed.

Industry scientists, however, figured out how to insert the Bt genes into the DNA of food plants (i.e., corn, soy, canola), turning the plants themselves into deadly killers for insect pests. The inserted GM Bt toxin is expressed throughout the plants, and so just by eating a leaf or stem, or any part of the plants, insects will die. The Bt toxin cannot be washed off because it is inside the plants. Certain natural Bt toxins have insecticidal properties, and are selective, killing the larvae of certain kinds of moths and butterflies and beetles. But there is strong evidence that genetically engineered Bt toxins lose their selectivity, leading to harm of nontarget organisms. For example, some insects that are helpful to farmers, such as lacewings and ladybugs, have been shown to suffer harm from exposure to GM Bt crops.[12] Even mammals have suffered adverse effects from being fed GM Bt crops,[13] which we will read more about in the next chapters.

The rationale for turning plants into pesticides (although of course the farmer isn't offered this wording by way of description) is that farmers reduce the need for *external* spraying of pesticides, and therefore lower their up-front costs. This is where the claim that GM crops reduce pesticide use comes from. However, this claim fails to take into account the rise in the use of insecticidal seed treatments on crops subjected to genetic modification since the introduction of GM Bt crops.[14] Insecticidal seed treatments are not taken into account in most calculations of insecticide use, which generally only measure insecticides sprayed over the top of the crop. It is important to note that since many Bt crops are also Roundup Ready crops, they are usually still being sprayed with (herbicide and fungicide) pesticides as well.

It is interesting that the way Bt toxin works in pests is by literally causing a leaky/punctured gut such that their gut bacteria poison the rest of their body. The mechanism for how this leads to leaky gut in insects is not the same as the mechanism for producing leaky gut in humans, as far as we know. What happens to Bt toxin in humans is unclear. One of the common claims is that because the pH of the insect gut is higher than that of humans (meaning it is less acidic), Bt will not be activated in the human gut. However, GM Bt toxin in plants is preactivated and thus does not require the alkaline gut of the insect to activate it.[15] We

Critiques of Studies Suggesting Safety of GM Foods

1. Compositional analyses of the GM versus non-GM foods only look at basic components (fats, carbohydrates, and proteins). If the GM crops' contents are in the normal range, they are considered equivalent to non-GM crops. More definitive methods of analysis (such as metabolomics) have found they are not equivalent.
2. When industries study GM versus non-GM crops, they often use genetically different strains of the crops rather than focusing on the same genetic strain with the only difference being the genetic modification.
3. Industry studies tend to evaluate only GM crops rather than GM crops plus their associated pesticides, thereby not mimicking real-life conditions.
4. Studies finding the GM food tested is safe often fail to ensure that the GM and non-GM crops were grown at the same time and in the same location, thus potentially skewing results.
5. GM crop studies generally exclude juveniles, but in their conclusions generalize for entire populations (and life course), thus they might misrepresent actual risk for juveniles.
6. Industry studies often fail to account for animal deaths in relation to normal attrition versus study effect.
7. Much of the data that regulatory agencies use to evaluate and approve new GM crops are neither peer-reviewed nor published at the time of evaluation. However, industry often publishes its animal feeding studies ninety days *after* the GM crop is approved.

8. Animal feeding studies on GM foods performed by industry and academic scientists generally last for a maximum of ninety days, which is not a long enough period to reveal long-term changes.
9. Studies concluding the GM food or crop tested is safe often fail to control for pesticide and GM contamination of the test and control diets. As laboratory rodent diets are routinely contaminated with pesticides, heavy metals, and GMOs, the resulting effects could mask any changes that occur due to the GM sample being tested.
10. Studies concluding the GM food tested is safe tend to dismiss changes found in the GM-fed animals as not biologically significant/relevant—an interpretation that is often disputed by critics. These conclusions often fuel reluctance on the part of US regulatory agencies to investigate possible health problems with GM crops and their pesticides.
11. The fact that funding by agroindustries for studies on GM foods often produces findings that are favorable to agroindustries should raise questions about bias.
12. Reports and studies on the safety of GM crops and their associated pesticides are often merely re-reporting results of previous studies (many of which are funded by industry) rather than generating new data.
13. Industry studies tend to report on gross parameters in study animals (e.g., organ weights) whereas new critical studies look at metabolomics (chemical fingerprints of metabolites of cellular processes), which give a more precise reading of differences.

also know that in one study, Bt toxin protein was found circulating in the blood of pregnant women and their fetuses and nonpregnant women, though it is unclear where it came from (the natural soil-dwelling bacterium *Bacillus thuringiensis* or GM Bt crops).[16] Again, we'll go into this more in the next chapter.

GM advocates consistently argue that there is no evidence that suggests Bt plant crops have any negative effects on human health. However, most of the studies that have been done to show safety of GM foods had until only recently been done in order to show substantial equivalence to non-GM crops.[17] This is not the same thing as studies of whether or not they are safe for humans. We have epidemiological studies of glyphosate's effects on animals and humans, but we don't have studies of the effects of GM foods. And, on the claims reported by industry that studies show substantial equivalence between GM and non-GM foods, there is much debate, with many studies showing substantial differences.[18] There is also a growing body of research that shows in animal studies the harmful effects of Roundup Ready GM plants, which we will also talk more about in the next chapters.[19]

Finally, it is worth noting that even many of the so-called "safety studies" of GM foods that have been done on animals are debated by scientists. This includes debates over questionable design, the length of time the studies were conducted, the age of the animals tested, and the composition of the feed used to study the animals. Scientists who question the results of industry studies point repeatedly to the way that some concerning results seem to be dismissed as "not biologically significant." This is before we turn to problems of what, according to critics, seems to be a pattern of industry manipulation of publication processes, ghostwriting of research reports, and pressuring regulatory agencies over suppressing negative data.[20]

More Regulatory Blind Spots: Protecting the Public versus Advancing Industrialized Food

If the basic science of GM foods is agreed upon, what is not agreed upon by a long stretch is whether or not these foods are safe for humans. In our experience, most scientists find the debate over the safety of GM foods to be without merit. The majority seem to feel the claims about the dangers of GM foods are spurious, whether or not they are actually familiar with the scientific studies.[21] Our position, simply by questioning the safety of these technologies and their associated pesticides, goes against the grain, but we join a growing group of scientists, educators, moms, clinicians, and activists who are voicing similar concerns.

To be sure, again, we are not arguing *against* uses of genetic engineering as a technology in and of itself. Indeed, many branches of biomedicine are exploring extraordinary things with such technologies, using cross-species genetic manipulations to grow or repair organs, to make new drugs, and to eliminate genetic diseases. We also note that scientists have even proposed the use of genetic engineering to design probiotics that could target specific problems of dysbiosis.[22] But it is important to remember that *those* genetic interventions are, and will always be, subjected to extremely rigorous testing on human subjects before being approved.

We are not suggesting that clinical trials are the *only* way to decipher potential risks versus benefits to new technologies (in fact, much of the medicine in the integrative medical world relies on technologies on the basis of clinical case studies and evaluations rather than large evidence-based randomized controlled studies). Still, the question of the long-term impacts of modifications to the food supply has never been subjected to the same level of rigor (e.g., human subject testing) when it comes to GM foods. This is because the standard that had to be met with these foods was so simple: "Are they substantially equivalent?" To answer this question, regulatory agencies took the companies' word for it. And as we mentioned in chapter 4, because food is not seen as a medical substance, it still doesn't have to be tested, even when it has been made to resemble some of our most complicated pharmaceuticals. This is a big problem.

So, the sad reality is that genetically engineered foods have never been and are still not tested for safety on *human subjects* before being introduced to our food supply. In the United States, the industries that make these crops need only to prove to the USDA that they are not plant pests or noxious weeds in order to obtain "deregulated" status.[23] Regarding food safety, there is a voluntary notification system whereby the companies inform the FDA that they are placing the GM food crops on the market under the assumption that they are generally recognized as safe (GRAS), and the FDA is supposed to evaluate the evidence accordingly which, as Druker notes, is inadequate.[24] That is, the FDA does not undertake its own safety tests of these foods on human populations or animals, but rather relies on industry studies.[25] Not surprisingly, animal feeding studies with GM crops that do exist have become a huge source of controversy in contemporary debates over food-health safety in both Europe (where substantial equivalence is used) and the United States (where GRAS indices are used).

It is also useful to remember that the EPA has very little ability to regulate the use of genetic technologies in agricultural industries, despite its appearance as a federal regulatory agency soon after Rachel Carson's exposé on DDT. As we said, the EPA regulates Bt crops as pesticides, but does not see them as risky to human health. The USDA regulates GM organisms only if they are thought to be, again, plant pests or noxious weeds—and, if perceived as neither, they get deregulated status.[26] In other words, unless the USDA decides that GM technologies are putting *existing* crops and livestock at risk, they cannot regulate the agrochemical industries or keep them from using these innovations. Since the industrial food and agriculture industries state that GM technologies are GRAS status, the USDA has no incentive to regulate them.

Again, the EPA *can* regulate pesticides, using the notion of no observable adverse effect levels (NOAELs) for pesticide toxicants in crops, essentially the level of toxicant that produces no adverse effects. But these levels are based almost *entirely* on industry-reported findings (mostly animal studies of the risks). This concept of "acceptable levels" is constantly being challenged by activists and has been since the era of Rachel Carson, who said (and we paraphrase) there are *no acceptable amounts of many of these pesticides*—many of which are still used today. Yet, there has been little to no progress in improving regulatory processes or limiting use of the chemicals.

The bar is very high for those who wish to get the EPA to ban toxic pesticides. The amount of effort required to produce enough evidence to go against the findings produced by industry is prohibitive for most non-industry-funded activists. In the end, the EPA is, and has been, largely ineffective when it comes to overseeing pesticides and food production.

Finally, even the FDA would not technically be interested in regulating GM foods unless it was convinced that the *toxic load* of these plant foods was unsafe. But, again, its data on this are narrowly focused on scrutinizing information produced by the agrochemical companies, which maintain that these foods are substantially equivalent to other crops already deemed safe for human consumption.[27]

The substantial equivalence analysis that is used by all these agencies is far too simplistic. It looks only at a few basic known components, such as fats, proteins, and carbohydrate levels, and states that they fall within the range of these components in non-GM crops of the same type. This type of analysis ignores unintended effects of the GM process on the crop, which can cause major changes in the profile of the types of proteins and metabolites that make up the plant. This was the issue raised by Belinda Martineau (one of the inventors of the Flavr Savr tomato).

The devil is in the details when it comes to GM foods; what is important is not whether, say, the total amount of proteins present has changed, but the amounts of different *types* of proteins, and similarly the amounts of different types of fats, carbohydrates, metabolites, and so forth. Only in-depth molecular compositional profiling will reveal if the GM transformation process, with the novel gene functions it generates and its inherent mutagenic DNA damaging effects, has resulted in significant changes in the food plant, including the potential production of new toxicants or allergens.

Currently, GM crop compositional testing as required by regulators and conducted by industry is not much better than what you might read on the side of the box of your breakfast cereal! By failing to demand a detailed, in-depth molecular profiling analysis of GM crops and foods, regulators risk missing crucial compositional changes, which might have health consequences. Furthermore, the FDA does *not* do postmarket analysis of these foods that end up on the dinner table. In other words, like the USDA and EPA, the FDA takes the industry's word for it that these foods are safe, or at least nutritionally the same as non-GM foods. Again, activists, scientists, and consumers strongly contest this.

As new technologies become available for gene editing, such as the CRISPR technology, new regulatory efforts are required. The US Coordinated Framework on Biotechnology appears to be the newest government effort to consolidate policy making on such things as GM technologies. This agency groups together and evaluates old transgenic genetic engineering with new gene-editing technologies that provide a more targeted way of modifying plant host gene function.[28] However, because offices like this are charged with covering a vast number of uses in agriculture, medicine, and biotechnology, and because they are often staffed by scientists and industry representatives who stand to profit from them, and thus have a conflict of interest, there are many questions about how likely such agencies are to set policies that err on the side of being overly permissive.

In the world of GM crops in the United States, the regulation (if any) often only occurs after grassroots opposition, organic farmer opposition, and filed NGO-driven lawsuits that succeed in very local ways, often only at the county level, where bans against GM crops are put in place.[29] Lack of regulation has become a major problem, with federal agencies tending toward laxity and bureaucratic evasion, leaving most regulation to occur only at the local level, county by county and state by state.

Even if there were some federal agency with sufficient jurisdiction in the United States, the question of *toxicity load* with the use of genetic modification and its associated pesticides is one of the more contested issues about them. While the makers of these foods continue to maintain that they are perfectly safe on the basis of their studies, researchers (mostly Europeans) undertaking studies today are showing results that call the industry's safety claims into question, although no studies have yet been completed on GM foods and humans. This is important.

The fact is, the public is already voting with their pocketbooks on these issues; vast swaths of the public already want labeling for GM foods and they want organic foods stocked in their supermarkets. Still, the conventional scientific and medical communities have not caught up with these trends and, indeed, remain skeptical of them. The gap between the widespread skepticism and widespread endorsement of the idea that we should be regulating, if not eliminating, the use of these crops is both shocking and frightening. Too often we experience what we call "GMO eye-rolling" when we bring up this issue. In fact, sometimes activists' vehemence can be as off-putting as blatant industry bias. It is important, especially in the medical community, however, to bridge this gap and understand how to use language and research to engage the skeptics' attention. We believe that if the reluctant scientific and medical constituencies were convinced to become engaged more deeply with these issues, things could change very rapidly.

To convince the skeptics, we, as medical professionals, need to delve into the science about these food crops, their associated pesticides, and the evidence of their safety (or lack thereof) in human health. We must combine clinical experience with emerging leading-edge science. Before digging deeper into how to do this, then, let's return to more of the clinical evidence Dr. Perro has gathered over the years that led her to question the safety of these foods.

Carlos: Into the Environment and Out of Autism

Carlos was a six-year-old boy from the Central Valley of California, right in the heart of a heavy agricultural center. He and his one-year-old sister were brought in to Dr. Perro's office by their parents, Sonia and Ernesto. They had seen many clinicians and therapists but had run into only dead ends.

Carlos was diagnosed with autistic spectrum disorder when he was two years old. His mother described him as having been sick for several weeks immediately prior to his eighteen-month-old checkup. Like many parents of children like him, his mom wondered if his diagnosis had anything to do with the series of immunizations he received, as his decline in health followed shortly after being vaccinated and, they feared, resulted in Carlos's sudden loss of speech and motor and other cognitive skills. Sonia talked slowly and deliberately about how, over a period of only several weeks after the shots, he lost all of his language skills as well as fine motor abilities. He became unaware of his environment and no longer laughed, engaged, or played with his sister. He would flap his arms (this is called *stimming*) and show violent behavior, such as hitting his preschool classmates. He seemed constantly agitated. Eating became impossible and mealtimes would go on for hours because Carlos became extremely picky and selective, refusing to eat most of what he was offered. He complained of a chronic stomachache and his mom noted that he was always constipated. Sleeping became a huge problem in their household because it seemed that Carlos needed less and less sleep and awoke frequently during the night screaming. The impact on the parents, Sonia and Ernesto, was obvious. They were distraught and at their wit's end. They felt as if they had lost the Carlos they knew.

Dr. Perro listened to everything the parents described. She noticed that even getting a detailed history involved Carlos's father taking Carlos out of the room so that he couldn't disrupt their conversation. The physical exam was nearly impossible because Carlos couldn't settle down. He was distressed and continuously screaming. As with many children she saw with autistic spectrum disorder, Dr. Perro focused on the gut.

She knew from Carlos's stomachaches and constipation that something was wrong with his digestion. She also determined that he had chronic inflammation of the gut, intestinal permeability, and dysbiosis based on laboratory analysis. She ran tests on his food sensitivities and noted he had extremely high levels of all IgG food antibodies, particularly to dairy and gluten. He had high levels of unhealthy bacteria in his gut and significant yeast overgrowth. His low digestive enzymes signaled that protein and fat breakdown were compromised. She thought some of his problems were related to his declining appetite and nutrition. She also found that Carlos had a genetic predisposition to difficulty with detoxification via assessment of his MTHFR genes. Additionally, she learned, using the Environmental Pollutants Profile urine test, that he had dangerous levels of chemicals and pesticides in his urine, including high levels of quinolinates (a breakdown product of phthalates) and organophosphate pesticides (the panel for glyphosate, a different class of organophosphate, was not available at the time).[30] She knew quinolinates were known to be neuroinflammatory, and that organophosphates were also linked to neurocognitive dysfunction.

Over the next two years, Dr. Perro worked methodically with Carlos's parents to change Carlos's internal and external ecosystem. This began with talking about toxicant exposures in their home environment. She immediately worked with them to develop a treatment program that would detoxify Carlos and simultaneously heal his gut. She had the family switch completely to an organic diet and to remove gluten and dairy. She managed his leaky gut and dysbiosis through a combination of homeopathic remedies (drainage and immune-modulating remedies), probiotics (high-level *Lactobacilli* and *Bifido* strains), and herbal formulas (to eliminate yeast overgrowth). She later used amino acids and antioxidants to detoxify and high levels of B vitamins to correct the deficiencies in his levels. She had the family run regular laboratory tests to evaluate the status of his nutritional deficiencies, yeast balance, and toxicant levels.

Working with kids who are on the autism spectrum can be challenging. In so many cases, one can do things to ameliorate symptoms, but depending on how long the child has had the diagnosis, it can be very hard to reverse the course of this disorder. Not all children with autism are alike, and clinical trajectories can vary widely. In Carlos's case, his transformation was dramatic over a two-year period. Despite the fact that he had struggled with severe autism symptoms from the time he was two, his symptoms were radically subsiding. His appetite improved and his constipation resolved early on. Then Carlos began to make eye contact with his parents and even begin to laugh appropriately. His arm flapping disappeared and, eventually, his sleeping pattern reverted to normal. By the time Carlos was seven, he was able to attend his regular neighborhood school with an aide. Improvements were not always steady, and occasionally there were small setbacks with illness or inadvertent divergence from his diet. But Carlos's parents were actually starting to believe their son could lead a normal life.

Another interesting aspect of Carlos's case was that his father, Ernesto, who was thirty-two when Dr. Perro first started treating Carlos, also benefitted from his son's therapy. When Dr. Perro met him, Ernesto had chronic renal failure and only 20 percent kidney function. He stated that it was "genetic" and his mom and brother also had the same problem, noting that his mom was on dialysis. That, too, could have factored into Carlos's problems, Dr. Perro thought, but what was amazing was that when the changes were made to Carlos's diet, the whole family switched to organic food. Ernesto didn't do the elimination diet or take any of the supplements, but he did switch over entirely to organic foods. He described the situation to Dr. Perro and said that because of the financial strain this put on the family, since organic foods generally cost most than conventionally grown foods, he no longer ate out. He limited his foods to what they prepared at home. Since they lived in a region heavily contaminated with pesticides, this switch proved even more challenging. He was diligent, though, and made sure to check labels and ask before he bought even the dairy and meats to be sure they were only organic.

Nine months later, Ernesto was very surprised. At his yearly appointment with the nephrologist, he found he now had 80 percent of his kidney function back and a notable drop in his elevated blood pressure. His nephrologist was also shocked. She was even able to take him off his blood pressure medication. Ernesto told his doctor that the only thing he had changed was to switch to an all-organic diet, wondering if that was what got him better. The nephrologist didn't think it was likely.

We hear this a lot. Many people, including many physicians, will dismiss the idea that organic foods are healthier options, and they will doubt that that alone could change debilitating conditions. Skeptics will say that there isn't sufficient research that shows organic food is better for health (and they are partially right; there isn't a lot). They will also point out that switching to organics prompts patients to improve their diet overall, and health improves from this, whether or not this improvement is specifically from *organic* food. But, in our opinion, eliminating pesticide-laden foods makes a *big* difference. Along with many others, we argue that eating healthier foods ultimately *must* mean eating organic in order to reduce the overall load of toxicants in one's body. The idea that this specific change might work to improve disorders that are thought to be intractable and irreversible (like Ernesto's kidney problems and perhaps Carlos's autism) is what is being suggested here. In other words, being nutrition-conscious means thinking about *which* foods and also *what is inside of* foods. We must pay attention to not just the nutritional composition of foods but also to how they were grown. We also must recognize that this is an issue not of individual choice but of public health. The provision of healthy foods should not be reserved for the well-to-do who can live in uncontaminated zones and buy uncontaminated foods.

Of course, Dr. Perro didn't just prescribe changes in diet for Carlos. Diet alone might have made a difference in Ernesto's health, but she gave Carlos a wide palette of treatments. All of these probably helped improve Carlos's health. Nevertheless, a cornerstone of any treatment for food-focused medicine is eliminating foods that don't support gut health, and this always means getting rid of foods doused in glyphosate, other pesticides, and those made of Bt. Without changing the dietary intake to solely organic, the other array of treatments won't hold. Without changing to organic, even the best of treatments and successes aren't, in Dr. Perro's experience, able to be sustained.

So, let's return now to the question we began with: What exactly is the evidence that GM foods, in particular, contain hidden toxicants that we have ignored for many years? Let's dig into the research, and the controversy.

CHAPTER ELEVEN

The GM-Food Debate: Controversy, Politics, and Truth

Much of what needs to be done is undoing what's already been done.

GM-Food Critic

Those who venture into the GM-food territory are met instantly with the reality of a huge gap between those who say there is ample scientific evidence to suggest our industrialized food production systems (and specifically GM crops) *are not* safe, and those who say there is ample scientific evidence they *are*. Even when some people across this divide agree that many well-known and commonly used pesticides are harmful to health, these same people frequently don't believe the same is true for GM foods. Our position is that GM foods are *the key ingredient* in the larger toxic pesticide problem, thus they cannot be separated. This, of course, is also hotly debated. We saw some of this debate in chapter 10, concerning criticisms of the industry's own science and the resulting regulatory blind spots that arise therefrom. Here, we will go into the politics of knowledge that have penetrated the debate over the positive evidence that GM foods are harmful to our health.

Some note that upward of 88 percent of the scientific and biomedical community feels the GM critics have got it wrong—that these foods and the pesticides that accompany them are entirely safe, and certainly safer than if we didn't use them. On the other side, however, similar reports note that the majority of the public disagrees with this scientific consensus on this topic. So, while 88 percent of scientists feel it is safe to eat GM foods, only 37 percent of the public feel this way, and 67 percent of the public believe scientists do not have a clear understanding of the health effects.[1] On top of this, nearly 90 percent of the American public support the idea of GM (or GMO) labeling, suggesting a very high rate of public suspicion of GM foods.[2] Is this a case of collective blindness and ignorance of the scientific truth? Or is something else going on? For an astute overview of the ways these politics get problematically constructed, we recommend Glenn Davis Stone.[3]

It cannot be overstressed that the specific debates over GM foods in industrialized agriculture are perhaps among the *most* controversial in our contemporary era. This story will be familiar to those already ensconced in the debate and the literature. But for those who are not, it is important to know this story in some detail. The story of controversy here resembles, depending on which side you are on, a myth of apocalypse and conspiracy perpetrated by antiscience activists or, if you are on the other side, a return to the drama of corporate-funded corrupt science hiding the truth about the harms of their products in order to continue to reap outsized profits. On one side, the debate is compared to the climate change debate (with climate deniers likened to GM critics) and, on the other side, comparisons are made to the previous era's tobacco wars (with agrochemical industries being likened to the tobacco companies that obfuscated, lied about, and fought the truth for years until the truth was outed by public outcry, persistent doctors, and scientists and, eventually, government investigation).

Today, it is virtually impossible to learn more about the science on the topic of GM foods without trudging through this murky and muddy terrain. For instance, one need only spend a short amount of time on the internet or in the annals of peer-reviewed publications to see how virtually every critical assessment of GM foods is juxtaposed to counterclaims that support their use. Critics of GM foods see a David versus Goliath battle, with activists, scientists, critics, and even neutral inquiring bystanders being drawn into combat with industry (and industry supporters), which, on the other side, has vast financial, political, and technological resources at its fingertips.

Critics of GM foods have taken the battle to the airways and mediascapes, where one can find a steady stream of evidence that points to the dangers of glyphosate, other associated pesticides, and GM foods themselves. Most of these sites and efforts are grassroots funded and supported. On the other side, one finds websites devoted to discrediting non-GM supporters and providing counterevidence from universities and government-sponsored agencies (such as the National Academies of Sciences, Engineering, and Medicine) that are weighing in positively on the safety of GM foods and their associated pesticides.

GM supporters are often quick to point out the lack of credentials of many GM critics (only some of whom are scientists), while the latter, of course, argue that the same is true of many GM supporters, who, additionally, are often being paid in some capacity by industries that profit from GM foods. Most GM critics point out that most of the so-called "independent" government-sponsored agencies (like the National Academies, above) are also made up of a majority of industry-supporting, industry-paid, or formerly paid experts.[4] There is a great deal of effort put into public shaming and character debasing on both sides. So, now that we know a little more about the political lay of the land (what some might call the *politics of knowledge*), what are the arguments we typically hear in support of or against GM technologies in food?

Exploring the Arguments in Support of GM Foods

At a minimum, pro-GM food advocates argue that:

- The agrochemical industries are providing food technologies that are perfectly safe for humans. Food security is no longer a problem because of these technologies, and there is ample science to back up both these claims. They argue that we need these technologies to feed the world.
- Genetic modification is a natural extension of the traditional selective plant-breeding tactics that humans have been doing with crops for thousands of years through selective breeding. Further, they argue that viral forms have modified the genome and thus the insertion of proteins into plant DNA has been happening since the dawn of life itself. The manipulation of this technique by humans, they say, is much the same as what has occurred naturally for eons.

- Using genetic-engineering techniques not only helps reduce loss to insect pests, infections, and weeds, but also improves upon the molecular and cellular qualities of the food crops through *enhancements* (e.g., reducing brown spotting, increasing the amount of vitamins, making them more fleshy, more drought resistant, with longer shelf-life). Again, this argument is used to claim GM technologies will solve our world hunger and nutrition-deficiency problems.

These pro-GM arguments are based on many decades of scientific reports from industry and industry-funded academics, as well as some independent research, that argue not only that GM foods are safe but also that most of the associated pesticides are as well. Again, the government's National Academies of Sciences, Engineering, and Medicine offers the most recent summary of the evidence on GM foods, including metastudies (that collect all the studies over multiple years and summarize their findings) of the so-called risks to health.[5] Not surprisingly, since most of these reports simply restate the findings of older studies, the latest reports from this group affirm conventional assumptions about the safety of GM foods and food production techniques, including pesticides. What is somewhat surprising, however, is that they also report that the benefits in terms of financial and crop yields, as a result of increased resistance in weeds, are no longer as clear.[6] In addition to the National Academies reports that attest to the safety of GM foods and GM-food technologies, there are other places one can find similar studies. For instance, the Genetic Literacy Project, the Alliance for Science, and multiple smaller institutes and centers on university campuses (that often have large agribusiness funding) provide arguments and resources attesting to the safety and necessity of these foods.[7] They note that there are peer-reviewed studies that focus on the safety of GM foods eaten by test animals. There are studies that focus on the safety of glyphosate in animals and humans. There are studies on the benefits to our food supply of using GM technologies in our foods. There are studies that argue nutritional equivalence between organic and nonorganic foods. Finally, there are studies affirming the lack of risk of GM technologies to our livestock, our crop resources, and our environment. Of course, there are also multiple opinion articles and blogs attesting to the lack of credentials of GM critics on these sites as well.

Questioning the Safety and Benefits of GM Foods

Those who question the safety of GM foods include a wide variety of people from many professional and nonprofessional walks of life. They are food activists, scientists, clinicians, parents, and neutral bystanders who find themselves having to wade through the controversies about food safety and GM technologies unwittingly. There is little disagreement among GM critics about nearly all of the flawed arguments put forward by GM-food supporters. Specifically, GM-food critics argue the following:

- Genetic engineering is definitely *not* a natural extension of the traditional selective plant breeding. Human insertion of foreign genes into plant DNA is significantly different in that it can create random new genetic expressions that these plants might or might not have ever developed naturally, even with cross pollination, selective cultivation, hybridization, or viral infection.
- Genetic engineering of crops and controlling the dependency of farmers on GM seeds create the possibility of stabilizing DNA in crops that become ubiquitous, and the resultant genetically uniform monocropping makes them more vulnerable than ever to pests, drought, and other threats that cannot be controlled.
- Even while increases in yields and profits might come from these crops initially, the cost of growing them increases because of the need to repurchase seeds each growing season along with new and improved pesticides on which the crops now depend. These problems actually harm poor farmers in the developing world rather than help them, thus posing huge risks of food *insecurity* around the globe.

- Questions about whether or not *enhancing* foods with genetic modifications is effective are still largely unanswered (for example, with genetically enhanced vitamin A–enriched Golden Rice).
- Questions about whether the nutritional quality of GM crops is better than that of non-GM crops grown organically are insufficiently answered, and what evidence we do have demonstrates that compared with organic foods, GM foods might be nutritionally different, especially when considered in relation to glyphosate's effects.
- Instead of reducing overall need for pesticides, GM technologies have increased the need for and use of biological and chemical products, particularly the use of the herbicide Roundup and, due to weed resistance, other more toxic herbicides.
- There is abundant evidence that GM crops can contaminate non-GM crops by cross pollination, even when the GM crops were only grown years before in field trials. This puts organic and non-GM crop farmers at risk of crop contamination.
- Most importantly, using GM techniques in food production has not been sufficiently studied to determine the safety for human consumption *sui generis* as well as in conjunction with the large amounts of pesticides with which they are now grown. No studies have been done on these crops in humans.

GM critics argue that there is ample evidence from the organic farming world that we do not need to use GM technologies or all these chemicals to grow our food. Reports from agroecology (a form of agriculture that focuses on imitation of natural systems and forests, with the goal of sustainable ecology) do not support GM foods. The International Assessment of Agricultural Knowledge, Science, and Technology for Development report on the future of food and agriculture (authored by over 400 experts, sponsored by the World Bank and UN) specifically does not endorse GM crops as a viable solution to world hunger and food security. Reasons this organization objects to GM crops are: lingering concerns over food safety; intellectual property rights on seeds, which would exclude poor countries; and "variable" yields.[8] Experts advising the World Bank also wrote that: "There are a billion people going hungry in the world today even though there is currently enough food to feed 14 billion people, well over the current world population of 6.9 billion, and even above the projected population of 9 billion in 2050." We feed enough grain to livestock to feed 3 billion people.[9] Also roughly one-third of the food produced in the world for human consumption every year—approximately 1.3 billion tons—gets lost or wasted.[10]

Thus, agroecology approaches that resist use of GM crops might put the current product lines of agrochemical companies out of business, but they will not starve the world. That is, if the agricultural model were refocused and used a more agroecological approach, we would see a drastic reduction if not elimination of agrochemical inputs, an increase in food availability (or, at the very least, not a decrease), and a world that is not, in fact, starving. An utter reimagination of our agricultural system is needed. In fact, it appears that GM foods do very little, and perhaps nothing, to solve world hunger problems. World hunger has much more to do with political and social inequality and poor distribution than food scarcity based on low yields. And it has nothing to do with the quality of foods produced.[11]

While there is good research demonstrating that organic yields can be higher, especially in drought periods,[12] it is true that organic yields are generally lower for commodity crops. However, there are pioneers who are showing successful large-scale agroecological, or regenerative, approaches, such as the North Dakota farmer, Gabe Brown.[13] Those who advocate agroecology to feed the world, however, point to increased food security (i.e., you can get more whole-food yield, such as fruits and vegetables, out of one acre of organic land than one acre of intensive monocrop commodity GM cropland). But accounting for yield and organics always has to be nuanced and qualified, as it all depends on what you are trying to produce, how, and to what end (feeding your community or generating cash exports). Meta-analysis shows organic food is up to 60 percent higher in health-giving antioxidants than conventional food. So clearly yield alone will not feed the world adequately and nutritional quality must be considered, too. We think that the arguments used by industry to date favor only one type of accounting, and that is not sufficient. If even a fraction of the money invested in agrochemical GM technologies, not to mention in federal subsidies for GM crops of corn, soy, and canola, was instead invested in distribution and support for organic food growing, the problems of hunger probably would likely be more readily solved than if we continue on the path of industrial food production.

Similar arguments are made about enhancements to foods using GM technologies. For instance, it is not certain that golden rice can actually reduce vitamin A deficiency, and in places where it has been experimentally tested, it shows unacceptably low yields.[14] We also have little evidence that making crops easier to transport or resistant to drought improves their distribution or availability, which again often has more to do with infrastructural barriers and socioeconomic inequalities.[15] GM crops don't solve these problems, but these problems make it so that GM crops are poorly distributed, often in the same ways non-GM crops are.

Without structural and policy changes, GM crops are subject to the same issues of lack of access, poverty, and infrastructural barriers that plague other foods. For instance, say a tomato plant is modified to enhance its shelf life. In theory, the tomatoes it produces can more easily reach communities in food deserts that don't have access to or are not close to farmland, right? Wrong. It's the distribution aspect (the lack of stocked supermarkets in certain locations) that determines food access, not changes in the food. It's also that even when organic food makes it to these markets, lack of money can be an obstacle to people buying them. These are different problems altogether, but they are seldom accounted for in GM promoters' claims that GM foods will solve hunger problems. We suspect that if organics were the only option, they could be supplied in ways that would be competitive with GM foods, even in food deserts.

Perhaps the most convincing argument by GM-food critics is that the so-called *virtuous* endeavor to use genetic modification to enhance food is not even relevant to the GM food that is actually grown and sold in the United States (and which, thereby, provides significant profits to GM industries). Only about 1 percent of GM technology falls into this category.[16] The other 99 percent of the industry's GM effort goes to the few crops that have little to do with saving the poor or food-starved world (soy and corn). Enhancements are not what time, energy, or money are spent on in the industry. The more one tries to verify these claims, the more these humanitarian rationalities seem like a rhetorical maneuver designed to make the GM supporters sound humanitarian in the face of opposition.

Beyond the current GM crops, there are new products and technologies emerging all the time, and the same questions arise about not only their safety but whether or not we truly need them to improve our food supply. These new developments can be broadly divided into two categories: those using gene-silencing technology based on a method known as RNA interference (RNAi) and those using so-called gene editing based on new CRISPR technologies. RNAi is used to switch off a gene function either in a GM plant, thus altering some characteristic (e.g., nutritional value, browning), or conferring insecticidal properties by switching off a vital gene in an insect that feeds off the crop—thus killing the insect. RNAi can also be used as an insecticidal spray during crop cultivation. These technologies are the next generation of engineering after "old-style" genetic modification.

Why should we be worried about these new techniques? Contrary to what was previously believed, there is now firm evidence that the molecules that mediate RNAi, small double-stranded RNA (dsRNA), survive digestion and can enter the body of the (animal or human) consumer. As a result, the dsRNAs might not only switch off the intended gene in the plant or insect but might also interfere with one or more gene functions in the body of the consumer, with potential adverse health outcomes.

The Arctic apple and Innate potato, which have been engineered to not brown upon cutting, entered the market in 2016 and 2017, having been produced using RNAi technology. Knowing that RNAi technology can have off-target gene-silencing effects, what potentially could be wrong with these products that can potentially result in negative health outcomes? First, unintended alterations in plant biochemistry leading to novel toxins can be produced, and second, unintended gene silencing in the consumer can lead to ill health. Neither of these health risks has been adequately taken into account by US regulators in considering market approval for such products. Indeed, the USDA has granted "deregulated" status to both of these products, which means that no safety testing is required for either, leaving the public unaware of their GM nature and at risk for any unintended effects.

In sum, new techniques of gene editing mostly involve either knocking out (destroying) or tweaking the function of one or more genes in the organism of choice (bacteria, plants, farm animals). Although a targeted modification of one or more genes can be brought about by this method, there are inevitable off-target effects; that is, unintended changes to host genes other than those intentionally altered will accompany the intended change. In the case of a food crop, this can lead to alterations in biochemistry resulting in the production of novel toxins. A variety of mushroom that was engineered to not brown on cutting has been produced by knocking out the function of an enzyme using gene editing. The question is: What unintended off-target gene effects have also been produced? Off-target effects are twofold. First, the intended change in a gene or genes can have unexpected outcomes. For example, changes in the activity of one or more enzymes can result in unexpected altered biochemistry. Second, off-target gene disruption of the editing procedure will result in changes to the organism's biochemistry. Both of these can result in production of novel toxins or allergens. The fact that the USDA has granted "deregulated" status to this nonbrowning mushroom means that none of these potential adverse outcomes need to be evaluated prior to marketing.

To date, the only GM farm animals destined for human consumption that have been approved for commercial use are salmon, which have been engineered with growth-hormone genes to enhance the rate at which they grow and thus more quickly reach marketable size. As escape of these GM fish into the wild is seen as inevitable, this development has raised major environmental concerns.

One of the helpful organizations working on bringing truth about the GM concerns to light is Friends of the Earth, which offers an excellent summary of the research from a critical perspective in its report *Spinning Food*.[17] The book *GMO Myths and Truths* also provides a comprehensive and well-researched summary of the debates over safety of GMOs.[18] Steven Druker's *Altered Genes, Twisted Truth* offers a thorough account of the industry's legal and regulatory histories in relation to GM foods. We offer a longer list of GM information and activist resources in the Resources list at the end of this book.

What is certain is that the average reader and the concerned clinician, who might be blinded by the science in all these studies, are both at a serious disadvantage in forming educated opinions about the safety and risks of GM foods. Indeed, if one goes to the internet and the scientific materials, truth sometimes feels particularly elusive when it comes to this topic. Nevertheless, clinicians do not have the privilege of not taking sides. They have to evaluate whose truths are more reliable and valid, sometimes even before the evidence base for clinical care has caught up with the laboratory science. Food-focused clinicians often side with the GM critics quite simply because that research helps them make sense of the clinical profiles and outcomes they see. Dr. Perro found herself deep in this literature when it became clear to her that her patients were experiencing symptoms similar to those researchers found in animals eating GM foods. She also found that simply getting her patients onto organic-only diets—meaning no GM foods or their associated pesticides—helped solve many of their problems right off the bat.

So, what is the scientific evidence that GM foods and their associated pesticides might be harmful to our kids' health? First, let's walk through some of the evidence that GM foods in and of themselves might be harmful. In chapter 12, we will focus on the evidence that their associated pesticides (or, more specifically, glyphosate) are also harmful to our health.

Animal Research on the Harms of GM Foods

Early on, a few scientists began to publish on the dangers and the risks of eating transgenic (GM) foods. One of the first things one learns about these studies is that nearly all of these scientists, after their findings were made public, were and are still attacked over their work.[19]

Let's consider one example: Arpad Pusztai, a Hungarian-born biochemist and nutritionist who spent thirty-six years at the Rowett Institute in Scotland and whose expertise was plant lectins. The research he conducted between 1995 and 1999 revealed that rats fed "GM potatoes had stunted growth and repressed immune systems, with a thickening of gut mucosa."[20] The transgenic crop he studied was the potato modified to contain lectin from the snowdrop bulb (*Galanthus nivalis* agglutinin, or GNA), a natural plant insecticide that, like Bt, was designed to protect the plant against insect pests (although it was incidentally learned that it also protected against nematodes, or worms). He did not set out to find flaws with this technology. In fact, he was surprised by his data.

In Pusztai's study, six rats were randomly allocated to each group and were fed diets containing either raw or boiled GNA-GM potatoes, parent potatoes, or parent-line potatoes supplemented with GNA for ten days. He found that the rats fed GNA-GM potatoes had thickened mucosal lining of the stomach with concomitant cellular hyperplasia, increased length of intestinal glands (crypt of Lieberkühn) in the jejunum, thinner mucosal lining in the part of the small intestines where it joins to the large intestines, and higher intraepithelial lymphocyte counts per villi. As the group of rats fed the parent-line potatoes supplemented with GNA did not have any of these same effects—that is, they showed the same results as a control group fed just parent-line potatoes, these findings clearly pointed the finger at the GM process and not the GNA insecticidal protein per se being at the root of the adverse effects observed in the GM potato-fed group.[21]

In sum, these GM potatoes seemed to be causing structural changes in the gut that the non-GM potatoes did not cause. Although we know that increased mucus from intestinal cells found in the stool can be a sign of inflammation and pathology (such as colitis), and that increased numbers of lymphocytes also suggest immune system activation, it is not clear what the clinical implications of the intestinal structural changes might have been in Pusztai's work, because further research to explore these findings in new studies was never done.[22] Pusztai was attacked and his work was buried. Indeed, tragic circumstances prevented Dr. Pusztai from following up his observations of the GM potatoes.[23] As a result of Pusztai's work, the particular GM potatoes he studied (GNA) are no longer available and were never brought to market. What is interesting, however, is how quickly his career was destroyed by the controversy around his findings.

Pusztai's public statements about the consumption of GM foods ("I wouldn't eat it," he said) immediately triggered massive attacks against him, including accusations of ethical violations for going public with his findings before publication, even though he was apparently authorized by his institution to do so. Within days after his public statement, the UK government, the Royal Society, and even the Rowett Institute where he worked launched an aggressive campaign against him. He was sacked by his institute, his research team was disbanded, and his data were confiscated. He was forced to sign a gag order banning him from speaking about the findings of his experiments under threat of legal action. His telephone calls and emails were diverted. He was subjected to a campaign of vilification and misrepresentation by pro-GM scientific bodies and individuals in an attempt to discredit him and his research.[24] Suspicious outsiders called in to question the attacks, and one investigation found that there had been a phone call from Monsanto to the then US president Bill Clinton, from Clinton to the then U.K. prime minister Tony Blair, and from Blair to the Rowett Institute.[25]

The tragedy of this episode, beyond the fact that Pusztai's career was destroyed by these politics, is that the GM crop industry and researchers were not stymied. Indeed, industries are still researching and developing GNA-GM crops. There is at least one 2007 study on GNA rice.[26] Studies like this, and the details of the controversy around them, seldom find their way into the hands of clinicians, especially if they are forcibly retracted, as the next case shows.

The second most well-known of attacks made against researchers who were finding dangers in GM foods is that of the famous European scholar Gilles-Eric Séralini, whose work, published in 2012, led him to report liver and kidney damage (one of the main causes of premature death in male rats) and other organ damage (pituitary damage in female rats) linked to Roundup-tolerant GM corn and exposure to even very small amounts of Roundup.[27] His 2007 study of rats fed GM maize already showed liver and kidney problems.[28]

Séralini was attacked on multiple grounds, including accusations that his work lacked statistical validity, that his use of tumor-prone rats showing tumors (even though it was a toxicologic study) was not necessarily from the GM food, and that he provided insufficient information about the procedures he used. As with Pusztai, the journal in which Séralini published his work came under fire for having published it. He was asked to retract his work, but he refused, noting that it had been previously approved by the peer-review process. Eventually, his publication was forcibly withdrawn by the editor of the journal (*Food and Chemical Toxicology*).

Séralini's study was subsequently republished by another journal.[29] The controversy and attacks against him were daunting.[30] The non-profit organization Sustainable Pulse reports on how industry scientists orchestrated the attacks on Séralini and his lab.[31] Still, if one were to simply read the most available media about this, it would be hard not to be suspicious of his work or not to think that those who support him are not qualified to evaluate his work and are driven by a spurious conspiracy against agrochemical industries.[32]

Controversies like this have led some of the scientists who are concerned with the results of the industry-sponsored studies to go back and scrutinize the results in those studies. For instance, in a GM study of three generations of rats fed GM corn, critical scientists point out that histological changes *were* seen—meaning the cells in the organ tissues showed changes—but they showed no differences in organ weight or body weight. The authors of this study therefore concluded there were "no significant health effects," even while calling for more study.[33] These pro-industry authors also left unexplored the significance of the fact that the Cry1Ab proteins (a form of Bt toxin) *did show up* in the rats' liver tissue. Results like these leave some investigators wondering what the definition of "no significant health effects" really is here.

There is a long list of researchers who have produced original scientific data on the risks of GM foods, following after Pusztai and Séralini,[34] including studies on the effects of glyphosate, which we will go into in more detail in the next chapter. As prelude to that, we'll discuss in more depth some of the risks scientists take to do work in this area by examining the work of Andres Carrasco, an Argentinian developmental biologist who published research in 2013 on the adverse effects (birth defects) of glyphosate in frog and chick embryos. He was also attacked by Argentine authorities.[35]

Like Arpad Pusztai, Carrasco was accused of unethical behavior for reporting his findings publicly prior to publication. He was also accused of conducting flawed scientific work, although his defenders argue that his work was rigorous and the attacks were largely based on the political implications of the conclusions he drew. His laboratory was apparently stormed by lawyers for the consortia of agribusiness companies in his home country of Argentina, followed by demands that his work be evaluated and he be dismissed. The fear that his findings would detrimentally impact the GM soybean industry in Argentina was apparently so great that the US embassy in Buenos Aires was motivated to become involved in the investigation and the punitive efforts that followed.[36] Carrasco was denied promotions even while he, like the other researchers, became something of a hero to public activists, scientists, and clinicians worried about industrialized farming as well as the role of GM technologies in this. Carrasco died of a heart attack a year later at the age of sixty-seven.

In the media aftermath of these investigations, the stories about these researchers are often publicly labeled as "affairs"—the Pusztai Affair, the Séralini Affair, and the Carrasco Affair. This debasing terminology lends itself to the ways in which melodrama becomes not just an artifact but also a driver of the science here, obscuring truth and facts in a sea of political conflicts. The consistent pattern of attack is striking insofar as it suggests that it is not simply motivated by scientific rigor (or that science has built-in mechanisms for self-correcting in and through peer review). Rather, as we will see, the pattern suggests deliberate and orchestrated efforts to target researchers who publish against GM foods.

The scientists we have discussed are only the most well-known in a much larger pool of researchers who, privately and some with unwillingness to be named, have been pressured to drop their research on the effects of GM technologies in foods. Sometimes this pressure has come from leadership within their universities as industry-supported (or supportive) scientists learned about their work and called attention to it. Sometimes this pressure has come directly from industry in the form of threats to withdraw funding for other research at the university unless such pursuits were dropped.[37] For these and other reasons, there is a growing group of scientists who have been deterred from work in this area.

Is it possible that the majority of public opinion and these few but committed scientists are deluded and industry supporters have it right? Or is it the reverse? Is industry really obfuscating the truth to protect its profits against stalwart investigators and public supporters who are right to question the safety of these crops?

For the curious clinician scientist, academic, or consumer trying to make sense of GM food sciences and finding words such as "affairs," not to mention the numerous other critical scientists who have been publicly threatened or harassed and unfairly criticized for their work,[38] the pursuit of facts can lead one to feel like Alice trying to find her way out of Wonderland. Truth slips away not simply because the science is too technical, but because as more and more information circulates and as more and more media translations of this work are put forward, it actually obscures what the science says. The bar is so high just to get to the point of comprehension of the field—so high for anyone who jumps into this territory and who might be sympathetic to either side—most people just walk away from it or refuse to get involved.

The experience of the intrepid novice in ferreting out truth in the GM versus non-GM debate is, we would argue, much like that of the patient who is not getting answers from her regular physician(s) while her symptoms persist, sinking in a churning sea of dead ends and failed treatments. Similarly, it might be like the physician who has reached the end of his therapeutic repertoire and still cannot figure out what is wrong with a chronically ill patient. What do most of us do when presented with a situation of indecision, of having competing routes to truth that leave clear decision making impossible? We go with our gut.

But what, exactly, does "going with our gut" mean here? It means paying attention to the kinds of studies that connect gut health to that of GM foods. That is, regardless of the larger debates over the merits and risks of genetic modification of foods and their associated pesticides, we can make sense of science here by focusing on the known qualities and characteristics of the foods that are eaten in relation to new knowledge about the microbiome, leaky gut, and chronic inflammation. Scientists today are looking at the gut in new ways, and this research is helping to reframe the debates about health, GM foods and their associated pesticides, and, specifically, the active ingredient in Roundup, glyphosate. Let's look at what we know about glyphosate.

CHAPTER TWELVE

Going with Our Glyphosate-Filled Gut

Glyphosate is the DDT of the 21st century. When future historians write about our time, and about our use of glyphosate (Roundup), they're going to write about our willingness to sacrifice our children, and to jeopardize the very basis of our existence and the sustainability of our agriculture.

Don Huber, PhD, emeritus professor of plant pathology, Purdue University[1]

Given the controversy over GM technologies, it is no wonder that contemporary researchers have tried to focus on a few key scientific concerns that have to do not with *all* GM foods, but with only the main ones currently on the market and in our food supply: Roundup Ready (i.e., glyphosate-tolerant) and Bt crops. In this chapter, we will focus on glyphosate, starting with the important questions: How much glyphosate gets into the typical body in those geographic locations where it is used, and is it harmful or harmless once it gets there?

As we laid out in chapter 11, there are industry reports on the safety of glyphosate. Many of these were done several decades ago, as genetic modification techniques were just starting. The potency of glyphosate as a weed killer goes hand in hand with the genetic modification to seeds that allows them to withstand the use of this chemical. Glyphosate has long been considered one of the safest weed killers available, and even now many agencies attest to its safety, such as the United Nations' Food and Agriculture Organization and the European Food Safety Authority. These conclusions go up against new reports that state the opposite, namely that glyphosate and/or its commercial formulations (such as Roundup), even in small doses over a long period of time, is harmful to health. We'll look at that evidence here.

Glyphosate Is Everywhere, Including in Our Bodies

There are claims and counterclaims about *how much* glyphosate is actually getting into humans and *how much* might be needed to produce negative health effects. Some scientists are concerned with the fact that previous studies do not account for the higher levels of exposure to glyphosate herbicides that are now being experienced in real-world settings. But, as we will see, apparently even small doses might have health effects.

In the United States, glyphosate use increased by a factor of more than 250fold—from 0.4 million kilograms in 1974 to 113 million kilograms in 2014.[2] One report noted that: "in 2015, US farmers and ranchers applied enough glyphosate to spray about three-quarters of a pound of active ingredient on every acre of cultivated cropland in the country. Levels of glyphosate . . . are rising in soil, water, food, and the atmosphere. People are being exposed through multiple sources."[3] Increased use of glyphosate is principally the result of increased cultivation of glyphosate-tolerant GM crops and the resulting spread of resistant weeds. Whereas prior to use of GM foods, plant crops might have been exposed to spray once, early on, as weeds were eradicated, with GM foods, farmers can spray multiple times throughout the life course of the crops. On top of the regular use of glyphosate to *grow* crops, we mentioned that Roundup is also being used now to *kill* (referred to as "desiccate") some crops, especially cereals such as wheat and oats, just before harvest, augmenting further use of Roundup and the pervasiveness of glyphosate in our ecosystem.[4] Thus, inquisitive scientists ask: If it is in plant crops and if more and more of it is being used to grow these crops, how much is actually getting into humans who are exposed to its seepage into the environment and who eat these foods daily? For a map of glyphosate's use in the United States, see the reference in this endnote.[5]

The EPA has set the safety levels for glyphosate in crops at different levels that can range from 0.1 parts per million (ppm) for peanuts to 400 ppm for nongrass animal feed,[6] the so-called maximum residue levels (MRLs).[7] GM proponents argue that these levels are appropriate for two reasons. First, they argue that glyphosate biodegrades in the environment (sometime after 4 but up to 190 days, and some studies suggest longer),[8] and it is unlikely to get into people in significant quantities through their food. (But we now know it does.) They also say that because glyphosate is soluble but chemically stable in water, even if it does get into animals and humans through food or water, most of it will pass through the body without much impact.[9] Consequently, GM proponents argue that most exposure/ingestion among humans is within regulatory-permitted limits and well below harmful levels. We will return to this later. First, though, let's look at how much is likely getting into the environment and, consequently, into human bodies in places where it is heavily used.

In fact, scientists concerned with the safety of GM foods designed to be sprayed with large quantities of Roundup (glyphosate) contradict what the GM advocates say. First, GM critics say that glyphosate gets into human bodies by way of rainwater, surface runoff, and leaching into groundwater. It does, in other words, persist in the environment. They also say that use of such large quantities of Roundup results in the absorption of toxic ingredients by way of the plant's surfaces and by way of the groundwater that collects these herbicides, thus it *is* getting into foods persistently, so it might then become absorbed into human bodies.[10] Widespread home garden use of Roundup also increases the likelihood that it enters the bodies of humans through household or neighborhood use as well. Because GM foods are such a pervasive part of the typical American diet, the levels set by the EPA for glyphosate in crops is inconsistent with the need to calculate total accumulation levels in the average consumer of these foods.[11]

Just how much glyphosate is getting into humans has never been studied until now. As a reminder, because glyphosate works by disrupting the shikimate pathway, research points to the likelihood *it is* having an effect on the microbiome, as well as on metabolic processes that show up in problems with organs, among other things, as we will see.

So, how much glyphosate is in our foods? A 2015 European report compiled by the Soil Association noted that glyphosate is actually found in bread that is produced from wheat and grains that use herbicides containing glyphosate. The average amount found for 2013 and 2014 was around 0.2 mg of glyphosate per kilogram of bread.[12] In one study that looked at twenty-four breakfast foods, glyphosate was found in ten of them. Specifically, it was found in: "oatmeal, bagels, eggs (including the organic variety), potatoes and even non-GMO soy coffee creamer. . . . The fact that it is showing up in foods like eggs and coffee creamer, which don't directly contact the herbicide, suggests that it's being passed on by animals who ingest it in their feed."[13] Knowing how many children eat nonorganic cereal for breakfast should set off alarm bells about their exposure to glyphosate via this route.

How much glyphosate is in humans? We know that glyphosate appears in higher levels in the urine and (some argue) in the breast milk of populations, and this is *not only in agricultural places where it is heavily used*.[14] For instance, one study in 2015 notes that glyphosate was found in the urine of 93 percent of the American public at an average level of 3.069 parts per billion (ppb). The regions with the highest levels were the West and the Midwest, with an average of 3.053 ppb and 3.050 ppb respectively, with children having the highest levels with an average of 3.586 ppb.[15] A recent ongoing study in Indiana is now reporting that 90 percent of pregnant women had glyphosate in their urine.[16] The grassroots organizations GM Freeze and Friends of the Earth Europe have undertaken similar studies. They tested the urine of 182 city-dwelling volunteers from eighteen European countries in 2013. Forty-four percent had urine containing glyphosate. Of the ten volunteers from the United Kingdom, seven out of ten had traces of the weed killer.[17] Finally, one controversial study showed glyphosate was found in the breast milk of sixteen out of sixteen German women.[18] However, there are reports that state glyphosate is not found in breast milk in some places.[19]

In sum, there is ample evidence that glyphosate does, in fact, show up in human bodies.[20]Given the fact that the Food and Agricultural Organization sets the allowable daily intake levels (ADIs) for humans at from 0 to 0.3 mg/kg body weight (or 300 micrograms per kilo of body weight),[21] we ought to know more about both what these allowable levels mean in relation to the amounts showing up in crops and in relation to human health. We are only now beginning to see research that explores what intake levels translate into in animal studies using new metabolomics research tools. We don't yet have any data for humans.

As we will see, most of these findings show reason for *alarm*, not dismissiveness. The possibility that glyphosate is showing up in breast milk should be doubly alarming. Children's capacity to detoxify and process chemicals is very limited, and the effect of glyphosate on rapidly growing cells is potentially profoundly damaging, as we see in studies of other pesticides.[22] Remember that pro-GM scientists continue to argue that if glyphosate appears in the urine of humans, this means that at most only about 30 percent is absorbed from any ingested product and this would put it well *below the daily allowable intake as well as any level that would make it toxic*.[23] But many argue that given this evidence, we ought to be studying the impacts of even small amounts rather than assuming anything.

In fact, current allowable levels in the United States are set but hotly debated. According to the US EPA, safe levels of glyphosate are up to 1.75 mg/kg body weight per day (mg/kg/day, or 1,750 μg/kg) using what's called the chronic reference dose level (cRfD). In contrast, as we mentioned previously, European rates are nearly six-fold lower at 0.3 mg/kg/day (300 μg/kg), (a level adopted in 2002). As of 2017, California is debating using a no significant risk level (NSRL) of 1,100 μg per day (for a 70-kg person), which is roughly 127 times lower than current levels set by the US EPA.

Defenders of glyphosate argue that the current levels are safe (and that California's levels are far too low), but critics argue the levels are far too high everywhere because there is no known safe level, as we will see. Keep in mind, these NSRL levels in California are set for determination of cancer risk, but not for the many other possible adverse health effects. Also remember that studies of how much glyphosate is actually in humans are based on urine samples that do not tell us how much is actually in the body, only what is being excreted. Finally, since the allowable levels are set for adults, not children, we simply don't know what safety levels should be for children. In other words, activists maintain that until we know this, we should be using allowable levels that are much lower than current standards (if not banning it altogether). To this end, some researchers are noting studies that already point to the need for lower allowable levels, and activists are using this research to petition for change.

Studies on the Impact of Roundup and Glyphosate on Health

New information based on animal and in vitro human endocrine studies (outside of the body in lab tests, which are not as ideal as in-body or *in vivo* tests) is showing that even small amounts of exposure to glyphosate can be harmful. One group of researchers found that glyphosate augments the growth of human hormone-dependent breast cancer cells.[24] The Séralini lab found that Roundup was toxic to human embryonic and placental cells.[25] Another research lab reports DNA damage in fish exposed to Roundup,[26] and one peer-reviewed study has been published in *Environmental Health* that shows the levels of glyphosate-based herbicides, which the general public are commonly exposed to in drinking water, altered the gene function of over 4,000 genes in the livers and kidneys of rats, indicating damage to structure and function.[27] Finally, we have new studies that show liver damage in laboratory animals exposed to even extremely low doses of Roundup.[28]

Specifically, research from Michael Antoniou's labs (at Kings College in the United Kingdom and at UCSF), using protein composition profiles (called proteomics) and small-molecule biochemical profiles (called metabolomics) for analyzing liver tissues, showed biochemical markers of nonalcoholic fatty liver disease (NAFLD) from ultra low doses of Roundup! His studies used 4 nanograms per kilo of body weight per day of glyphosate. These glyphosate doses of Roundup were 75,000 times below European Union–permitted and 437,500 times below US-permitted levels of daily ingestion. This is the first study to provide a *causative* link between an environmentally relevant level of Roundup ingestion and a serious disease.[29]

Antoniou's group also notes that in these studies Roundup is shown to inhibit the action of liver enzymes responsible for the breakdown of toxic substances that get into the blood (even from medications).[30]

Finally, they also point to toxic impacts from adjuvants that come in glyphosate-containing products.[31] Adjuvants are additives that are put into glyphosate herbicides along with glyphosate. Their purpose is, for example, to enhance the toxicity of glyphosate to the weed by enabling the glyphosate to penetrate into the plant tissues.

There are challenges in this work. Some research argues that glyphosate, in and of itself, is not toxic because it cannot be absorbed by cells, but that the other additive ingredients in glyphosate-based herbicides and the biodegradation product of glyphosate (AMPA) are shown to be toxic to animals.[32] In fact, most toxicity studies done by industry are apparently done on glyphosate alone, rather than on glyphosate-based herbicides like Roundup. However, in order for glyphosate to enter plant cells, it must be used in conjunction with adjuvants that help break down the cell membrane. So, studies of glyphosate alone are incomplete.

Another challenge to research in this area is that it is difficult to decipher how much harm comes from GM foods alone versus how much comes from GM foods and their associated pesticides (especially those sprayed with Roundup), and although there have been animal studies that have successfully done this, many studies done on animal populations simply consider both at once. In fact, this might more accurately offer insights about what is happening in humans, since we are exposed to *both* GM foods and their associated pesticides because they were designed to be used together. From animal studies like these and from other laboratory research, the data suggest that GM foods plus associated pesticides show higher toxicity than GM foods alone. Séralini's research showed that GM corn alone (that is, the corn grown but not sprayed with Roundup) was toxic, and more recent studies show that GM maize is not substantially equivalent to non-GM maize.[33]

Some of the research that looks at impacts of glyphosate-based pesticides is revealing that they can disrupt normal microbiome populations.[34] Dr. Judy Carman, a physician and nutritional biochemist in Australia, for instance, found impacts of GM Roundup Ready and Bt toxin crops in animals. She took "168 just-weaned pigs and fed them a typical diet for the piggery, containing soy and corn, for 22.7 weeks (over 5 months) until the pigs were slaughtered at their usual slaughter age. Half of the pigs were fed *glyphosate-tolerant (Roundup Ready) soy and Bt maize* (the GM-fed group) for the whole period and the other half of the pigs were fed an equivalent non-GM diet (the control group)."[35]

Carman's results showed the level of severe inflammation in stomachs of the pigs fed the GM diet was markedly higher than that of those fed the non-GM diet. Specifically, pigs on the GM diet were 2.6 times more likely to get severe stomach inflammation than control pigs. Males were more strongly affected. While female pigs were 2.2 times more likely to get severe stomach inflammation when on the GM diet, males were 4 times more likely to get inflammation.[36]

One of our biggest concerns about glyphosate that is directly related to nutritional health is, as mentioned, that it was patented as an antibiotic in 2010 for microbial infection and parasitic control of various diseases.[37] We now know much more about both the beneficial and nonbeneficial effects of long-term ingestion of antibiotics on the microbiome. The concern is that as long as glyphosate remains in food, and especially at increasing levels, it will have effects similar to those of other antibiotics on the gut microbiome. In other words, previous studies that looked at glyphosate-based herbicides as low-toxicity alternatives to previously much more toxic substances were not aware of the large role played by the microbial populations in human gut health; studies of glyphosate's impact on cellular and organ damage alone are insufficient to the task of deciphering overall impacts on metabolism.

We know from one study conducted on the microbiota of chickens in vitro, for instance, that Roundup results in the beneficial bacteria like *Lactobacilli* dying off and the more pathologic bacteria such as salmonella and *Clostridiales* species (such as *C. difficile*), which are resistant to glyphosate, proliferating.[38] This study shows these biotic effects occurring at levels of exposure (.075 ppm) that are higher than those seen by Antoniou's lab, which showed liver toxicity effects at 4 nanograms per kilo of body weight. Even if the antibiotic effect appears to require higher levels of toxic exposure, these amounts of glyphosate are already being seen in human populations. We need more studies that explore what ingesting glyphosate does to the digestive pathway in humans, and at what levels effects (like those seen in pigs or chickens) might be also seen in human guts. Beyond this, we need to know, if disruption of our gut microbiomes is occurring, what effects, if any, this might have on other things the microbiome does, like produce folate and amino acids.[39]

Another proposed pathway for disruption of healthy digestion by glyphosate is that it is a chelator, which means that it binds tightly to metal ions. These ions include iron, copper, cobalt, zinc, manganese, and calcium, among others.[40] The concern here is that glyphosate might chelate these important ions in plants and in animals or humans that have ingested the chemical, thus making the ions unavailable to the body. In fact, one report notes that cows fed a diet containing glyphosate were found to have lower levels of copper, selenium, zinc, cobalt, and manganese in their bloodstream. It is not known how these lowered levels affect the health of these cows, or whether similar phenomena could be happening in humans with subsequent health effects.[41] Dr. Perro has also noted extremely low levels of crucial metals (magnesium, manganese, zinc, and calcium, for instance) in her chronically ill child patients, although whether this could be due to glyphosate exposures remains unknown. Urine testing for glyphosate has recently become commercially available for members of the public, but unless physicians suggest they do so, it is unlikely people will use it.

There are correlative questions about the additional "inert" ingredients in commercial products such as Roundup that augment the toxicity of glyphosate. AMPA is a metabolite of glyphosate and POEA is an adjuvant that is deliberately added to some glyphosate herbicide formulations—it is a surfactant. POEA creates holes in plant cell walls that allow glyphosate to penetrate cells. One of the key fears is that because this chemical works by destroying lipid-containing membranes (like a detergent), it could also destroy these membranes wherever it goes in the body, including those that protect the brain. Indeed, studies have shown that adjuvants, especially the POEA class, are highly toxic in their own right and that commercially used formulations such as Roundup are far more toxic than the stated active pesticide ingredient (glyphosate).[42]

What all this work suggests is that if these things are happening to livestock and poultry that eat food laced with glyphosate (and its adjuvants), then it is possible that the same thing or something similar will happen in humans. This includes effects that occur not only in the digestive tract, but also in the blood, in organs and tissues, and in the brain. Could it be that breaking down the lipid or fat lining that creates the blood-brain barrier leads to inflammation in the brain? Considering the rise in neurocognitive problems among children in the United States today, this seems like a fruitful area of inquiry. We already know that many toxic pesticides affect neurology and cognition, but what about the more subtle forms of pesticide exposure that come with the pervasive ingestion of glyphosate and its adjuvants?

In sum, although we don't have reliable studies on the impact of GM foods plus pesticides in humans, studies on animals point to the need for more reliable research. What we do have in terms of human studies is frightening but insufficient. One of these is the study cited previously from Indiana that found that 90 percent of pregnant women had glyphosate in their urine, but more importantly, it noted that higher levels of glyphosate appear to be correlated to shorter-term pregnancies and lower birth weights for newborns.[43] There is no explanation of causal pathways at work here, and one cannot assume that glyphosate is responsible for these outcomes. We also cannot assume that glyphosate levels correlate directly to ingestion of GM foods (as glyphosate exposure comes from many sources). However, given what we already know from animal studies, it should not take a leap of imagination to recognize that glyphosate (and the foods that it was designed to work with) might play some role in poor health outcomes, and that some of this glyphosate is coming from its use with GM foods.

What we already have, to date, is a consistent pattern of research showing toxicity in animals from GM foods and/or their associated pesticides, from the original work of Dr. Pusztai to the present work of Dr. Antoniou. There are consistent, reproducible findings over the last fifteen years of kidney and especially liver toxicity in laboratory animals fed either GM corn or GM soy, even if it is still not clear what component of these products (that is, associated pesticide residues, the GM transformation process, or both) is the cause of the observed adverse health effects. Evidence of liver toxicity from these foods and/or their associated pesticides, specifically demonstrated in the work of Dr. Séralini and the work of Dr. Antoniou, should be put in conversation with the fact that some 25 percent of Americans now suffer from a type of liver disease (NAFLD). Further, evidence from the livestock and poultry fields makes a strong case for the negative impact of GM foods and glyphosate on the gut microbiota. While there are surely numerous pathways to liver pathogenesis (that are not alcohol related), and there are many reasons for gut microbial disruptions (including pharmaceutical antibiotics or other foods that change gut composition), we would argue that GM foods and pesticides need to be explored as possible pathogens as well. Greater scrutiny of the appearance of GM foods, pesticides, and their residues in our foods and the rise in these disorders pushes research on the quality of our food to the top of the list. The existing evidence from contemporary research should leave little room for controversy on this.

Moving toward this goal of recognizing possible toxicity (on many different fronts), glyphosate was identified as a probable carcinogen by the World Health Organization in March of 2015, based on a review of toxicological and epidemiological studies by the International Agency for Research on Cancer (IARC).[44] In July 2017, the State of California also used the IARC report to place glyphosate on its list of 800 carcinogenic chemicals.[45] This report, not surprisingly, has been called into question by other agencies and agrochemical industries that continue to sell Roundup Ready seeds and glyphosate-based herbicides.[46] As mentioned, this is what California's proposed no significant risk level under Prop 65 was based on. Even the US National Pesticide Information Center, a collaborative center between the University of Oregon and the US EPA, states that chronic long-term exposure can cause health effects, and concurs with the IARC report stating glyphosate is a probable carcinogen.[47] The EPA's National Primary Drinking Water Regulations lists kidney and reproductive problems associated with high level long-term exposure to glyphosate. Why any regulatory agencies continue to support the high rates of glyphosate use for GM crops (not to mention newer and more toxic pesticides), even after the IARC report, leaves much room for speculation about the possible influences of industries that profit from these products. The IARC report was, of course, contested by industry.[48] Even without new research (building on previous contested studies) about the carcinogenic potentials of glyphosate, there appears to be ample reason to label this chemical as dangerous for human health.

One question that arises frequently when we talk about the possible effects of long-term exposure to glyphosate is this: Why, if we have all been so exposed to this product for so long, aren't *more* people sick? That is, if we are now getting reports of saturation of high quantities of glyphosate in human populations (especially in the United States), why aren't *all* people sick? The truth is, if you consider the population as a whole, we all are, in fact, sick. Our rates of multiple chronic diseases, including exploding rates of chronic disorders like nonalcoholic fatty liver disease, diabetes, Crohn's, colitis, and the list goes on . . . , should be read as a sign that our collective health is, in fact, in decline. The fact that not all people are sick at the same levels or in the same ways might have more to do with individual capacities to clear toxicants, genetic predispositions, and combination effects of exposures. But the fact that not everyone is sick in the same way should not be a reason for dismissing concern.

Is Glyphosate Changing the Nutritional Quality of Our Foods?

Up to this point, we've explored some of the evidence that glyphosate enters human bodies and that it is probably harmful to health for a variety of reasons that are related to the health of the microbiome, the presence of this chemical in the bloodstream, and its possible chelating effects. We should also, though, be paying attention to the other ways that pesticides, including glyphosate, might be affecting the nutritional quality of the foods we eat.

Research among progressive organic farm projects notes that plants that have absorbed high levels of glyphosate actually have lower nutritional value as compared to plants that have not been sprayed with Roundup or other glyphosate-based herbicides.[49] We know that plants grown organically do have more micronutrients and far less pesticide residues and *heavy* metals (mercury, lead, and aluminum, for instance) than nonorganic plants.[50] One study suggests that glyphosate handicaps the plant's own defense system by eliminating the need for the plant to produce phytoalexins (antioxidating substances produced by a plant in response to a pathogen).[51] Phytoalexins might provide key micronutrients that expand the gastrointestinal microbiome when ingested.[52] The evidence that glyphosate changes the nutritional quality of foods is added to the evidence, mentioned in the last chapter, that GM foods are themselves substantially not equivalent to non-GM foods, as one study of Roundup Ready maize has shown.[53]

Similar questions are asked about the soil. Is the soil being depleted of nutrients and is its microbial population disrupted the same way animal guts appear to be because of the chelating (microbiome-killing) activity of glyphosate? At least one report has shown damage to soil because of glyphosate—namely, reduced activity and reproduction of earthworms in soil sprayed with glyphosate-based herbicides, coupled with undesired increases in nitrates and phosphates that increase risk of leaching or surface runoff of these nutrients into groundwater.[54] Here, we could revisit our questions about the symbiotic model of health, in which external environments need to be healthy in order for the foods to be nutritious and, in turn, to feed (or otherwise supply) a healthy gut. If glyphosate is having an effect on the species that inhabit the soils where our foods are grown, what effect is it having on the foods, but also on the health of the ecosystem that we need to keep our guts healthy as well?

Questions about GM foods are generating research that, speculative in some quarters but definitive in others, is starting to change the conversation. In sum, we know that there are strong indications that GM foods and their pesticides are probably health altering for humans. At a minimum, if glyphosate's properties as an antibiotic enable it to disrupt the soil, the food, and the microbiome, then why wouldn't we assume it was contributing to dysbiosis, and to conditions that exacerbate (or possibly create) leaky gut (and enable unhealthy bacteria to colonize)? If the gut is leaky, in turn, could it be that these same toxicants and bacterial by-products (endotoxins) from the gut are getting into the bloodstream, and into the brain? Based on patterns and evidence generated from clinical experience, these are the pathways that Dr. Perro feels are at play in many of the sick children she sees.

Does Eliminating GM Foods Alone Improve Health?

Animal-feeding observations have actually already begun to affirm suspicions that gut-related disruptions could be a direct result of eating GM, pesticide-laden foods. One such layperson study by a pig farmer, Ib Pedersen, for instance, showed that switching to non-GM food supplies reduced his pigs' need for antibiotics by 66 percent.[55] This supports the notion that GM foods (and their pesticides) create an antibiotic environment that is unhealthy for normal gut bacteria in pigs. In this case, the pigs stopped getting diarrhea once they switched off the GM foods; they also showed reduction of bloating and ulcers while their milk production increased. They subsequently further reduced reliance on antibiotic medicines. Similar effects were seen in their piglets that, on GM foods, had uniformly chronic diarrhea and mortality at roughly 30 percent, both of which were eliminated after the switch to non-GM foods. The insight here is that once the GM foods are eliminated from the diet, the gut remains healthier and is able to resist other kinds of infections, which, in turn, results in lower need for more antibiotics.

In another study, this benefit (of reduced antibiotic dependency) seems to come from removal of glyphosate alone. A German study tested oral remedies to modify gastrointestinal microbiota of dairy cows whose urine indicated high levels of glyphosate ingestion from their feed. Like many industrialized dairy cows, the cows in this study were constantly dealing with problems of botulism, requiring use of antibiotics. Testing simple remedies using charcoal and humic acids (organic constituents of soil called humus) that would reestablish healthy microbiota, these dairy animals had much improved health and significantly reduced levels of glyphosate in their urine.[56] If cows are dealing with chronic problems of gut dysbiosis on diets that contain large amounts of glyphosate, shouldn't we be studying whether something like this might also be true for humans?[57]

There are a few studies on humans of the effects of organic (non-GM) foods that have been grown without use of toxic chemicals. Urinary levels of glyphosate are significantly higher in people on conventionally cultivated foods compared to those eating only organic.[58] Another study showed that shifting to an organic diet for even as little as a few days to a few weeks significantly lowers dietary exposure to organophosphate pesticides based on urine analysis.[59] Such studies, in and of themselves, point to the need for eating only organic foods, even before we get to the specific explanations of *how* these products might harm human health. The fact is, increases in use of pesticides go hand in hand with both increases in use of GM-food technologies and increases in the levels of pesticides ingested by humans, including glyphosate. These foods and pesticides are now part of both our bodily and environmental ecosystems.

The Pesticide Escalator: How Much More Can We Take?

Particularly problematic, are the increased numbers of new pesticides that are now needed to protect Roundup Ready and other GM crops because more and more weeds around them are resistant to glyphosate. What has happened is that as weeds have become more resistant to glyphosate, farmers require use of other new and more potent pesticides that work in conjunction with glyphosate. Roundup will achieve obsolescence soon, as weed resistance to glyphosate grows too large for it to be effective. This is already occurring, and new products are being rolled out and used before they undergo what critics would consider adequate toxicity testing.

An example is the 2014 decision by the United States (the EPA) to approve Enlist Duo, a new combination herbicide comprising glyphosate plus dichlorophenoxyacetic acid (2,4-D), which was formulated specifically to combat herbicide resistance. It was marketed in tandem with newly approved seeds genetically engineered to resist glyphosate and 2,4-D. The EPA anticipated that a three- to sevenfold increase in 2,4-D use would result.[60] Keep in mind, 2,4-D is one of the weed killers used in Agent Orange.[61] The EPA revoked the approval for Enlist Duo in November 2015, presumably on the basis of new information of its toxicity, but in January 2017, Enlist Duo was registered again for use in thirty-four states on Enlist cotton, soybeans, and corn.

The fact that the EPA states that Enlist Duo is safe for infants, developing fetuses, the elderly, and more highly exposed groups (such as agricultural workers), but provides no information about the studies on which these safety claims are based, leaves room for a lot of unanswered questions. Moreover, many of the new pesticides are combination pesticides that are meant to be used with preexisting formulas (like those that contain glyphosate). Many safety rulings for new combination pesticides are based on the previously accepted safety standards for formulas already registered for use; therefore, they presume safety rather than testing for synergistic effects that might be harmful.

Another pesticide now used to combat weeds that are resistant to glyphosate is dicamba, which is an organochloride herbicide, a derivative of benzoic acid. Dicamba (and 2,4-D) are hormone (auxin) mimics and they kill weeds by hugely increasing the weeds' growth rate until they outstrip their nutrient supply and die. In order to protect crops against dicamba, scientists have figured out how to insert a gene from a soil bacterium (*Pseudomonas maltophilia*) into the DNA of the crops on which dicamba is used. This bacterial gene encodes for an enzyme that converts dicamba to another compound, 3,6-dichlorosalicylic acid, thus protecting the crop, and thus enabling it to survive being sprayed with the herbicide. Studies of the safety of this pesticide are reported in much the same way as they are for other pesticide and herbicide residues, in rather confusing (if not alarming) terms and in reference to their allowable toxicity levels.[62]

As we write, a new generation of GM crops and herbicide mixes is being produced. Known as the Xtend system, the plants (soy and corn) are engineered to withstand being sprayed with both dicamba and glyphosate, in an effort to deal with the massive glyphosate-resistant weed problem. Thus, although technically containing old ingredients, it is a next-generation product that, along with other new chemical and GM technologies, will likely replace the use of Roundup alone at some point, and resistance to use of these chemicals is already happening on a state-by-state basis.[63] The new generation of insecticide GM crops that are designed to overcome Bt resistance are those based on RNA interference (RNAi) employing short, double-stranded (dsRNA) molecules. These dsRNAs are used to target and switch off a vital insect gene and kill it. The dsRNAs can be either sprayed on the crop like a classical insecticide or engineered into a GM crop.

We should all be concerned by both the fact that studies are not being done for these new combinations of pesticides and the possibility that so-called regulatory safe levels for these chemicals might not be safe at all, since only high, unrealistic doses are tested by industry in support of regulatory approval. Modern science tells us that very low doses of pesticides can affect human health more than higher doses, yet these very low doses are not tested or assessed for safety in the regulatory process.[64] In addition, only the stated active ingredient (e.g., glyphosate) of any given pesticide is tested for safety by industry and assessed by regulators, even though no active principle of a pesticide is used alone. All pesticides of all classes (herbicides, insecticides, fungicides) are always used along with added ingredients (adjuvants) in commercial formulations, and these in combination have been found to be almost invariably more toxic, according to in vitro studies, than the active ingredient alone.[65]

The fact that hardly anyone is researching levels at which these chemicals show up in children's bodies adds to the senselessness of the system as it now stands. Children are *not* small adults. Levels of "safe" exposure to a chemical pollutant determined in adults *cannot* be extrapolated to be the same in children, who have a very different degree of chemical sensitivity.

Other strong pesticides are continually being brought to market for use with GM crops every year. Newer technologies that speed up the invention of new genetic modifications (such as the aforementioned gene-editing technologies) will add to the speed at which new kinds of chemical combinations can be devised to kill weeds and pests but not crops. Genetic engineering both creates the need for ever more potent forms of chemical warfare and provides a means of continually altering the plants and fertilizers and pesticides that are needed to ensure crop survival in this toxic milieu. We see this reaching crisis proportions in areas where there is a high level of spraying for experimental research on crops, including GM crops, and high levels of drift, such as in Hawaii.[66]

The concern among GM-crop critics is that the spraying of pesticides in conjunction with genetic modifications that allow for the use of these pesticides results in an arms-war type of race to defeat the weeds and pests faster than they can develop resistance. As more toxic formulas are devised, the genetic modifications of the plants must also be modified. A vicious cycle of demand for more genetic modification and ever more toxic pesticides gets set in motion. Regulatory agencies trying to keep up with these new toxic tactics for food production can barely track the data collection on animals (if and when it is available), which predominantly comes from the agroindustry, much less the data on how much is getting into the food supply and into human bodies (again, if it is available). As we have seen, regulatory agencies are simply not positioned or willing to take meaningful action.

The fact of rising amounts of new and more toxic pesticides in foods might make the problem of glyphosate seem small. In fact, glyphosate is still one of the most prevalent of all pesticides. As we have argued, just getting a handle on the facts about *this* pesticide is challenging, given the conflicting debates in the science and across industry and activism domains. However, given what we do know, we have ample reason to be worried about glyphosate harm, and the anxiety should only rise from there as one tries to fathom the newer and more potent armaments now being designed for sustaining our industrial food system. We are not naïve enough to suggest that organic food supply systems would not also face challenges from resistance and pests, but we would argue that if even a small portion of the effort and resources now devoted to agrochemicals and GM foods was put instead toward organic farming solutions, we would likely see solutions that were healthier than what we have now. There are researchers and organic farmers who are trailblazing and succeeding here, not to mention the local and slow food movement. These cumulatively show a different path toward sustainable agriculture. We should be paying more attention to them rather than chastising them for being "anti-science."

Are Our Children a Living Science Experiment?

The lack of studies on GM effects on humans is partly a result of the way this research gets done. It is very hard to control the diet of humans so that they are solely exposed to GM versus non-GM foods. You cannot dissect the bodies of human subjects the way you do biopsies on laboratory animals in order to see what the study effects are. Doing biopsies (on livers or intestines, for instance) on living subjects (particularly children) is possible, but it is extremely difficult. Ethical guidelines make it difficult to study the effects of toxicants on living human subjects. Getting biomarkers, such as in fecal matter, is difficult and expensive. This research overall is costly and it is not easy to find independent funding sources. Finally, independent research on genetically modified foods is inhibited by the fact that the companies own the patents on these seeds; independent scientists find it difficult to obtain GM seeds for their research. Ensuring that non-GM test foods are actually non-GM is also difficult.

Some critics argue that we should not have to do research on the impact of GM foods on humans for the same reason we do not do studies of any of our non-GM foods on humans. We simply don't test most of our foods. As is the policy with the FDA, the only time we do is when an outbreak occurs that can be tied to a food (e.g., salmonella, *E. coli*). But without these triggers, we assume our foods are safe. As we have seen, since GM foods are assumed (by regulators) to be substantially equivalent to non-GM foods, the assumption is they do not need testing.

But what if we thought that our industrial foods were causing an epidemic? What if we were seeing a wave of chronic disorders that could all be tied to chronic exposure to chemicals that we were ingesting in our foods? Wouldn't we then want to test our foods to see what they were actually doing in our bodies? This is the main question we pose.

In this chapter, we have shown that research on the microbiome in humans, and new omics (e.g., genomics, proteomics) research that looks at a variety of biomarkers associated with toxic chemicals, is available. The growth of basic science and clinical science research on disorders like leaky gut and the biochemistry of pesticides in the human body are also key to this effort. These approaches, though currently available only on animals, could soon give us clues as to not only what pesticides do but what the GM foods themselves do in intestines and other physiological and organ systems in the human body.[67] Given the evidence we already have, we call for more research on the links between GM foods and patterns of chronic exposure and ill health.

Even with a growing body of laboratory science, we are still a long way from having the necessary data to drive changes in clinical guidelines. The American Academy of Pediatrics has a Council on Environmental Health (COEH) that studies environmental issues of relevance to children's health. This council publishes resources for the evaluation and treatment as well as the prevention of toxicity in children from pesticide exposure. It recommends buffer zones around high-spray areas. Even so, support for the prevention of pesticide exposure in our most vulnerable populations has not drifted, if you will, into efforts to figure out how all of our children are at risk of exposure through foods, or what chronic exposures are likely to look like in different forms of ill health. In other words, the recognition of these risks has not translated to advice that can be embraced by clinicians in any practical way.

When progressive clinicians are confronted with a steady stream of children who are suffering from serious digestive problems, they are faced with a dilemma because they do not have the tools they need. Given the strong possibility that toxic-filled foods are contributing to dysbiosis and leaky gut, it makes sense, even if only on a precautionary basis, that a first step toward repairing the gut would be to eliminate root causes of gut problems. When Dr. Perro does this, most kids get better. In the first chapters of this book, we talked about children who were sick with gastrointestinal problems, allergies, asthma, and autoimmunity. In the chapters that follow, we'll explore chronic disorders affecting the brain or neurocognitive systems.

CHAPTER THIRTEEN

Can Getting Rid of GM Foods Improve Mental Health?

Sometimes food makes it worse.

MOTHER OF MIKE,
a fourteen-year-old patient

The promise and prospect of food-focused medicine are that simple changes in diet can improve the health of kids. This should not be a surprise. What will be a surprise to many is how many of our foods are *not actually healthy*. Foods cannot fix everything, nor clearly are they the *only* source of all of our kids' health problems. As we have said, most chronic health problems are complex, with complicated and multiple causes and multiple avenues of pathogenesis. Still, foods are a key ingredient in dealing with any disorder, regardless of its complexity. We argue that eating healthy foods, at a minimum (as opposed to eating foods drenched in toxic chemicals), is the most important starting point in healing the gut.

This is particularly true for kids with cognitive problems. The list and range of chronic cognitive issues that doctors are presented with today are vast. The list includes autism spectrum disorders, ADHD, developmental delays, and complex psychiatric issues such as bipolar disease and eating disorders, all of which are on the rise among our children. Dr. Perro sees kids who are having specific nervous system disorders such as sensory-processing disorders, which include visual or auditory processing, as well as chronic headaches such as migraine headaches.

Frequently, by the time Dr. Perro sees these kids, the families have already been offered a series of tests to rule out serious issues such as tumors, congenital or genetic disorders, infections, autoimmune disorders, or problems secondary to trauma. But, after these problems are ruled out, they are usually offered few treatable diagnoses. If they get diagnoses at all, they are often psychiatric, even if symptoms are very concrete and physical. Even when they give one of these diagnoses, child psychiatrists seldom consider the possibility that there could be an underlying metabolic, intestinal imbalance or toxic exposure that might be exacerbating, or perhaps contributing to, cognitive changes. Foods hardly ever come up in the causal thinking about neurocognitive problems.

For kids who present with psychiatric or behavioral problems, the first line of therapy is usually psychiatric drug therapies. Kids with ADHD are often put on Ritalin or Adderall, and children who present with pediatric-onset mood or psychotic disorders are often put on antipsychotics or antidepressants, even before they have reached puberty. In fact, we don't know what causes many of these problems, even if we know that some drug therapies *are* able to reverse or modulate the symptoms, especially of psychiatric and behavioral problems. To be sure, some families *are* advised to change their child's diet, such as reducing sugar with hyperactivity, or even treating with B vitamins for mood disorders. A few physicians also recognize that some kids with mood or cognitive issues also improve when they are taken off gluten and dairy. But it is shocking how often children are offered only strong pharmaceutical therapies for psychiatric, cognitive, and behavioral problems across the board. We would argue that no matter what drugs are needed or used for these problems, treating kids for dysbiosis and leaky gut at the same time usually helps them immensely.

The proposition here, to be clear, is that beyond the typical gut problems we see in kids, a wide range of neurocognitive problems, even those starting in utero that do not have a specific genetic cause, are *usually helped by changes in diet in some way, with an organic diet being a central ingredient in the medical arsenal.* We also argue that even when there are genetic causes for a certain disorder, improving the quality of the gut and of digestion will often help with the body's ability to manage these problems, including the absorption and effective uptake of pharmaceuticals. Take the simple notion that many medicines work better if the lining of the digestive tract is able to properly digest and absorb them.

Efforts to clean up their guts can and will produce beneficial effects for these children's brains, no matter how damaged they might appear. In some cases, there might be improvement such that the child can return to activities that were previously impossible, including immersion in a regular classroom. Sometimes, these kids can get off the drugs altogether. In other cases, creating digestive health simply augments the health of a child who might need to stay on drug therapies. Mike, a teenager from a suburb in Northern California, is a good example of this type of patient.

Mike: A Complicated Kid with Complicated Problems

Mike was a fourteen-year-old who lived with both of his parents and four siblings in a middle-class neighborhood. When he was about ten, his parents noticed severe behavioral changes that got him into trouble at home and at school. He would have loud outbursts. He started fights with his brothers and sisters, as well as with other kids. These were not normal boyish behaviors; Mike got so violent sometimes that his mother had to call the police. In one episode, he even threatened her with a knife. Over the course of his behavioral decline, his school put him on probation and, after a final serious outburst in which he threatened another student, they expelled him.

Mike's parents, Jim and Linda, were traumatized by the changes they saw and the cascade of their otherwise healthy son into what appeared to them to be a kind of madness. Their close-knit family was shaken to the core. They thought they were doing all the right things: Boy Scouts, church every Sunday, plenty of sports and plenty of food, including daily family dinners. In fact, foods were the last thing they worried about. Everyone in the family was a little overweight, they said, but they assumed this was a portion-control problem, not a problem of the *kinds* of foods they were eating. The people in their family looked like most of the people in families who lived around them. They never imagined that the foods they were eating could be related to Mike's sudden behavioral and mood changes.

We spoke with Mike and his family after he had been seeing Dr. Perro for several years and had become, in their words, "his old self" again. Mike described himself before having Dr. Perro as his clinician: "I yelled all that time, kicked holes in walls, punched holes in walls, and my parents needed to find something to help me calm down, to help me regulate myself. I was crazy." His calm demeanor and clarity of insight about his own behavior while we were talking to him were far departures from the things he was telling us about who he once was.

We gathered around the family living room, and they told us the full story. Mike narrated, but Jim and Linda also chimed in to clarify points and timelines, and to tell us details about pieces of the story. Soon after his behavioral problems started, Mike said, his parents sought help from a neurologist. His mom was told by this one doctor, he said, that his behavior sounded extreme, and although it was not initially off the spectrum for a young guy, it was clear he needed help. That doctor, Mike said, put him on a patch—an ADHD medication called Daytrana (a drug that has since been recalled).

That medicine worked a little, but it caused rashes where the patch was, and it made Mike extremely irritable. His dad added that he felt it wasn't really working. When he'd come off the patch, Mike's behavior was even worse. So the doctor added another drug, a second kind of ADHD medication. That medicine caused severe headaches; they were so bad that Mike couldn't study in school. Finally, that physician recommended a different doctor, a psychiatrist.

The psychiatrist put Mike on several more drugs. At one point, he was on the ADHD medication, an antidepressant to help him sleep, and an anxiolytic (antianxiety) drug to help him calm down. His dad recalled that instead of getting better, things only continued to get worse. His behavior was ramping up more, he was more and more irritated and aggressive, with more verbal outbreaks. He would get picked on at school a lot, and because he had a loud voice, he was usually the one who would get reprimanded, even though he was not always the person starting the fight. His dad was working several hours' drive from their home with a big commute, and it got to the point where he didn't feel safe leaving Mike at home with his mom. Mike was getting more and more violent.

The psychiatrist tried several *more* drugs and, as a result, Mike developed a pretty severe jaw tic. That again only made his situation at school worse. He also felt like one of the drugs was so strong, he had trouble staying awake. He was so groggy that he couldn't get out of bed. He missed swim practice because his mother could not rouse him. He'd fall asleep in class.

At this point in time, because of his earlier violent episodes and now his chronic falling asleep, Mike was expelled from school and began being home-schooled by his mom. Linda and Jim hoped to get him stable so that he could rejoin his regular class the following fall. Linda recalled feeling pretty helpless during this time. She described how they were going deeper and deeper into the medicines, but he wasn't getting better. He was, they all agreed, getting worse.

She said one time when she was trying to get Mike out of the car at school and he refused, he instead pulled a whole jar of Nutella out of his backpack and began to eat it. She had to get help from the school office to get him out of the car. And he only did so screaming and kicking, jumping around the car, honking the horn. She described how sometimes when they were driving he would threaten to open the door and jump out, even while they were speeding down the road. He refused to be obedient. "I was like a raging madman," Mike said. Linda said it scared her. Later that day, they had the episode where he threatened her with a knife and she had to call the police.

Linda described her growing frustration with her son's psychiatrist. First, she said, she called Mike's pediatrician and told him about all the medications he was on. That doctor thought that the number of drugs seemed excessive. She also described how this psychiatrist had at one point pulled him *off* all the first drugs he was on, cold turkey, and then started him on some new ones. That also seemed wrong to the pediatrician. He advised her to talk with the psychiatrist about reducing the number of drugs overall. Her experience with the psychiatrist was frustrating for other reasons, too. She said he tried to tell her that Mike's problems were all her fault. "It was amazing," she said. It wasn't what our culture was doing or what the family was doing even . . . it was all *her* fault. She was tearful as she told the story. "I had done so much to help him," she said as she listed the home-schooling and her ceaseless efforts to find the right doctor. She tried every way possible to engage him. And then this doctor told her to not be "indulgent" with him, and to punish him more severely for his bad behavior, as if his problems were a simple matter of her poor parenting!

"It was insulting," she said. All that put her on the course of trying to find alternatives. Her path to Dr. Perro began when she saw something on *The Dr. Oz Show* about how kids with ADHD were getting help from alternative doctors, and she thought maybe she could find someone like that. She looked up who was covered by her insurance and found Dr. Perro.

When Mike finally met Dr. Perro, things were really falling apart. His family was living in daily fear of him. His dad said, "We just didn't know anymore who the real Mike was. He was so jacked up on so many meds."

Dr. Perro listened to their stories. She remembered Mike's face was white and pasty, and he had significant truncal obesity, an ominous type of fat distribution signaling a possible metabolic disorder. She referred to his appearance as "doughy," a problem of not just being overweight but also of long-term nutritional deficiencies and toxicity. She saw a child who was really sick and a family in crisis. She looked at the list of medications he was on and asked Linda and Jim if they knew of a different psychiatrist or doctor near their home who would work together with her, and with them, to get Mike off the meds.

In the end, it would be a nine-month journey.

First, Dr. Perro used homeopathic remedies to help Mike detox as he came off the medicines. She also had Linda do a food inventory, to keep a diary of what Mike was eating and what the rest of the family were also eating. She ran multiple tests. While waiting for the food-sensitivity tests and reports on his toxic levels, she started Mike on prolonged gut-healing protocols, using remedies that were aimed at improving his body's ability to detoxify, as well as probiotics and different cocktails of nutrients. All this was started as he weaned off the psychotropics, slowly and one at a time, over a period of months.

It was a bit of a revelation to the family to learn how many of Mike's problems seemed to be related to his food sensitivities. Jim, Mike's father, recalled the experience as like having a light go on for the first time. First, they found out that Mike was very sensitive to peanuts—a huge shock to the family because they ate a lot of peanut butter. In fact, Mike was sensitive to a large number of foods, with heightened antibodies showing up after he ate carbohydrates, almost all grains, and dairy, but especially after peanuts and legumes.

Mike described his diagnosis:

> You know how there's levels of allergies where there's high allergy. Well, I was at the one just below the one where you would need an EpiPen. If I had been eating peanuts and thought I was allergic to them, it wouldn't have been such a problem. But my dad and I are big peanut fans. We used to get these big salted roasted peanuts. And we would eat them every day. On my breakfast toast: peanut butter. For dinner: peanut butter. On my pancakes: peanut butter.

Mike's dad echoed this when he told us that he used to make this meal called the Daddy Rollup—place a tortilla in a pan, brown it up in butter, and add peanut butter and peanuts and roll it up . . . the Daddy Rollup. It was so good; they all nodded. Shaking his head, though, he added that he now realized that he, too, was likely sensitive to peanuts and to all the legumes. He loved refried beans on his tacos every Sunday. Their normal eating habits were all wrong, Jim said.

Linda also recalled that, originally, they thought Mike's problem was with gluten. And she tried to get rid of that, too, and dairy. But when she homed in on the peanuts, it seemed to be the major trigger. Most of his outbursts would come after eating peanuts or other nut butters they had in the house, including sesame butter, almond butter, and cashew butter. They were all triggers.

When Mike's reports came back, they learned that his stool showed evidence of dysbiosis. What worried Dr. Perro the most, though, were his blood results that had a very elevated insulin level and high hemoglobin A1C that portended insulin resistance. In other words, he was prediabetic. She told them that if they didn't fix his metabolic problems, he would become diabetic. She advised getting all the junk food out of the house. The family heard this and went into action.

"I can't tell you how much resistance I got," Linda said. Linda's cupboard was full of carbohydrates and sugary foods, many of which were made with or covered with nuts. She used to shop at Costco, and would come home with flats of donuts, cookies, cereals, crackers, chips, and tons of premade foods from the frozen foods sections. None of it was organic. Over the course of the year she eliminated these things from Mike's diet, and they successfully got Mike off all the drug therapies. It took months and months of detox remedies and gradual decreases in the meds. But they really saw the difference once they fixed his diet.

Linda and Jim both described being initially fairly clueless about how the foods they were all eating might be creating health problems. "All the sugar, and carbohydrates. That was one thing," Linda said. But she never paid attention to the "organic" food labels. Linda described trying to make the shift in foods and eating habits. But she got resistance from her other kids. They wanted the same diet they'd always had. They told her that it wasn't hurting them, so why should they have to change? It didn't seem fair to make everyone in the family change their diets, so despite the fact that she saw the changes in Mike, she would lock up the foods that Mike couldn't eat in the kitchen pantry. This was the sugary foods, the peanut butter and Nutella, the peanuts, the potato chips, the glazed sweet pastries and cereals, and crackers. They ate lots of pizza, packaged brownies, and white bread, and Mike was denied all of these while his siblings continued to eat them.

Mike's older brother, David, came in at that point and he joined in the conversation. He told us that, unlike his brother, he could eat these foods and not "go crazy." But it was clear that even Mike's brother, although clearly mentally sharp, was pretty seriously overweight and certainly didn't look healthy. In fact, comparing them just on the basis of appearances at that point in time, one might likely conclude that Mike, despite his behavioral history, was much healthier than his older brother.

The focus of David's narrative was on Mike. He talked at length about how before Mike got well he had to sneak his own Oreo cookies into his room so that Mike would not get them. Occasionally, one of the siblings would leave the door unlocked and Mike would find it irresistible. He'd "go in for the kill" and eat as much as he could. These episodes turned him, in his brother's words, "into a monster." He would get totally out of control. His father affirmed the description. They were all living in some fear of his outbursts. As long as Mike stayed off the foods, David said, he'd be fine. In fact, he was pleasant. David described him as normal. But if Mike got the sugar, the peanut butter, the Nutella, he would get out of control.

Dr. Perro found Mike's case perplexing. It was hard to believe that Mike could be that reactive to foods. Although many of her patients had food-related problems, the severity and degree of emotional lability in Mike were astounding. She witnessed the behavior herself on his visits. All indications pointed to food as a culprit. So, she recommended Mike go on an all-organic diet that included high-fat foods, animal proteins, fruits, and vegetables, excluding dairy products, grains, sugars, and legumes. Her reasoning was that this diet would force his body to burn fats rather than carbohydrates, which she knew had been used successfully in children with other neurologically based issues such as seizure disorders. His diet also excluded foods that showed up in his lab tests as ones he was sensitive to. She hadn't seen it used for patients like Mike, with mental health issues. Still, she thought it would help. It worked. As long as he stayed *off* the foods he was sensitive to and the carbohydrates and remained strictly *on* the Paleo diet, he did well. Still, David clarified that even since Mike got better, he would occasionally get into these foods and they would make him crazy again.

We asked Mike why, if he knew they were so bad for him, would he keep eating these problem foods. He shrugged and said that people can have only so much control sometimes. "I know it is bad for me, and sometimes I can't help it. It's like a relapse," he said. "An addiction. And sometimes it is just too hard to resist."

At fourteen, Mike was a healthy, talkative, calm, and slim kid, and it was hard to imagine how hard this journey must have been for this family. Mike had a lot of hobbies that had been put on hold when his health declined. One of these was hip-hop dancing. He described loving his dance class and how all the girls flirted with him. As he got sicker, he became more removed and disconnected from the other kids. He told us, "I got more and more shut off. I lost a lot of friends. I was unable to connect with people. I was acting as if I could not even control my emotions. I'd say anything and everything would come out of my mouth. I didn't even care. I would see my mom crying and I wouldn't even care."

Linda and Mike both talked about how Dr. Perro had literally "saved his life." The changes they made through her treatment made him "normal" in the sense that he was in control of his emotions, he was no longer prediabetic, his insulin levels and hemoglobin A1c were now at normal levels, and his ability to connect with family and friends restored. However, although it was a success story, Mike's struggles did not end there. Over the course of the next year, Dr. Perro would get periodic calls from his mother, Linda. Mike kept relapsing, resulting in suspensions from school. As before, he was fine if he stayed off the problem foods, but when he ate them, he became emotionally unstable and lost control. Linda asked Dr. Perro to vouch for him with the school, to give them assurance that he was healthy enough to go back. Dr. Perro talked with Linda about the fact that she couldn't do much to help him if he couldn't change his eating patterns. She also talked about how there might be an underlying psychological profile that made impulse control hard for Mike. He might have an issue that would not resolve, in other words, no matter how otherwise healthy he was. Dr. Perro thought that in cases like this, if there is a serious psychiatric problem, a drug regimen might also be needed. Figuring out which drug might help him was the trick, and even then, keeping to the diet that was healthy for him was critical. Sometimes you have to consider a combined approach, she told Linda. His diet can keep him pretty healthy, but if he can't control himself, he might need some more help. She recommended they find another psychiatrist who would be willing to work with Dr. Perro in collaboration.

Many of Mike's problems had been caused by his ingestion of foods that were bad for him. His diet had been poor by any standard, loaded with sugar, carbohydrates, foods that had many calories but little nutrition and with nuts that his body apparently had a hard time digesting. Mike had been deficient in many nutrients that Dr. Perro documented in a nutritional laboratory assessment. All of the normal things his family ate—the pizzas, donuts, pastries, crackers, cereals, cookies, and jars of peanut or other nut spreads, in many ways a typical American diet—were loaded with nonfood substances (preservatives and sugars). They were also full of wheat, soy, and corn ingredients that were genetically modified or grown under conditions of heavy pesticide use.

Compromises to Mike's digestion perhaps reached a cataclysm at puberty when his adult hormones began to kick in. Why was Mike the only child to have these severe symptoms? They were all eating the same things, living in the same food environment. This happens all the time; one child out of several has problems while the others do fine, or at least better than the one who gets really sick. But all were unhealthy, even by conventional medical standards.

One theory is that Mike, perhaps because of his own predispositions incurred by genetics, epigenetics, or an early exposure to antibiotics as a kid, had a gut that was already impaired at an early age. His problems might have been from the sugar and carbohydrates alone. But it was also likely his problems were related to the fact that his gut was not healthy. His steady diet of contaminated foods probably made his gut very leaky. Perhaps because of his diet his dysbiosis became worse than that of his siblings. Perhaps because he had dysbiosis *and* ate a lot of gluten, and sugar, unmetabolized food molecules and other toxicants from his foods caused low-grade chronic brain inflammation. Perhaps some of these toxicants chelated key minerals that were crucial for optimal functioning of his brain. Perhaps some of the pesticides he was exposed to had a direct impact on his body's ability to produce neurotransmitters. Perhaps, in addition to any or all of these, pesticide residues might have acted as endocrine disruptors that created or augmented hormonal imbalances. Any, or even all, of these might be at work.

We wouldn't rule out the possibility that Mike had an onset of a serious underlying mental disorder. But dysbiosis and leaky gut might have helped push him over the edge, making a problem he was predisposed to even worse. Figuring out his gut problems, his food sensitivities, and repairing his digestion improved Mike's health dramatically. Undoing the damage stemming from his digestive problems turned him around.

It also seems fairly clear that other family members benefitted from changes to their diets. Mike's dad lost forty pounds by eventually following

Mike's diet. The family's tendency toward being overweight and veering toward being prediabetic suggested a need for dietary overhaul. In cases like this, Dr. Perro felt that it was just a matter of time before other family members would also be experiencing the effects of these dietary impacts if they stuck to their high-carbohydrate, high-sugar, high GM–food diet. Because the rest of the family kept eating questionable foods, they all probably had mild cases of leaky gut and dysbiosis, even if they were not yet experiencing the full-blown effects of these conditions.

It is hard to distinguish between the benefits of switching to a low-carbohydrate, low-sugar, and no nuts/legumes diet and those of one that is all of these things plus only organic. The fact is, just getting rid of high-fructose corn syrup and the grains and carbohydrates of highly processed, packaged foods is healthy in and of itself. However, switching away from these foods nearly always also means getting off the corn, soy, canola, and wheat products that they are made of that are simultaneously GM foods. So many of our food products are made with these GM ingredients now and, without labeling, it is difficult to avoid them in any of the packaged foods one finds at the grocery store. One wonders if Mike would have improved less, or not at all, had he just shifted to foods that were not packaged but also not organic. Either way, in getting off the packaged foods, he probably reduced his load of toxicants significantly, and perhaps this would have been sufficient. What we do know is that because switching to organic also means eliminating most of those packaged food items, it helps.

We believe that the switch to an organic diet improved Mike's digestive system and, consequently, the nervous system. This treatment can't solve all problems or even, in some cases, solve them in full, but it can help a lot, especially in conjunction with other therapies. In the next chapter we will look at another case of the connection between the gut and the brain and the benefits of getting gut healthy by getting off GM foods and their associated pesticides.

CHAPTER FOURTEEN

Can Autism Spectrum Disorder Be Improved by Way of Gut Health?

You know, just changing the diet makes a huge difference. Even for kids who are not autistic—kids with ADHD or anything—they can all do so much better on the right foods . . . once we got her detoxed, and the foods she was sensitive to out of her system, she started to come back around.

THERESE, mother of Sami,
diagnosed with ASD

Is it possible to halt or even reverse the course of progression of even the most mysterious of disorders, such as autism spectrum disorder (ASD), by making changes to the underlying physiological systems that contribute to a healthy brain? We saw, in chapter 6, that new research on the microbiome is pointing to important links between gut health and brain health. We know that there appear to be links between digestive disorders, such as IBS and chronic diarrhea or constipation, and mood disorders, such as depression and anxiety. Scientists have posited something called the enteric nervous system, by which interactions between nerve signals, gut hormones, and the microbiota of the gut shape cognitive processes. So what about more serious cognitive problems, such as ASD? Is there a way by improving gut function and gut health to treat this intractable and devastating disorder? We'll explore more about the multiple and complex issues of autism, but before going there, let's hear from another family about their experience with autism, or ASD.

Sami: The Progression from Autism to "Normal"

Sami was diagnosed with ASD when she was about two-and-a-half years old. Her mother, Therese, described realizing that Sami was losing behavioral, social, and physical milestones before the doctors diagnosed it. She had four kids and knew the normal progression of speech and physical development. When her fourth child, Sami, shifted pretty much overnight from being able to speak in coherent phrases to being completely unable to form words, and then started flapping her arms (stimming) in frustration over not being able to find the words, Therese began to panic. "She'd say, 'Dora the explorer, Mommy, outside play . . .' And then all of a sudden it was as if she couldn't say it. She would say 'Daaaa . . . Daaaa' and she'd just stand there flapping her arms," Therese told us the story as if she were still fighting that same battle with the events that unfolded.

Her pediatrician didn't think it was anything to worry about. In fact, she said there wasn't any need for Therese and Sami to come in to the office. But Therese knew something was wrong and when she Googled "speech regression" and "autism" popped up, she became hysterical. When she finally got into the pediatrician's office, her worst fears were confirmed. Sami was diagnosed with autism spectrum disorder.

Like a lot of mothers, Therese had a hard time not tying the symptoms to Sami's immunizations. She told us the symptoms began just after Sami had a series of vaccinations—four of them all at once (measles, mumps, rubella—or MMR—and chicken pox). She felt that even if Sami was predisposed to autism, the vaccinations seemed to be a trigger for her. Right after that, Sami started spinning and flapping, and her speech declined. She just kept going on this downward slope after that. Her doctor assured Therese that Sami's vaccinations had nothing to do with it, but Therese wasn't sure. It seemed crazy that she could have a totally normal child one day and the next, "pop," and suddenly she was not normal. It wasn't like she was just oblivious to the signs of it before then, Therese said. It was as if her child had been taken and replaced by a new one.

Therese's first stop was with an autism specialist. She ran a lot of tests and found out that Sami had mercury toxicity. Therese told us, "Sami also had two genetic defects. She was unable to metabolize stuff. The doctor tested all this. I don't know what else. Deficient in her supplements, leaky gut." They began treatments for detoxing Sami and it helped. She didn't completely improve, but it helped. Therese also found a DAN (Defeat Autism Now) doctor who worked with them on several fronts. Eventually these changes helped a lot, and Sami actually started speaking again. Therese attributed the improvement to three things: detoxification, gut healing, and vitamin B12 supplements.

Therese reasoned that if the onset of symptoms in Sami was sudden, it must have been triggered by something. Therefore, the solutions were going to be things that undid the damage from those causes, possibly restoring her to as close to the state she was in before it started. She described how one doctor at the specialist hospital told her that this was just the way Sami was going to be for life. "You are just going to have to accept it," he said. In response, Therese said, "No. If she's 40 percent functional and I can get her to 60 percent, then that's where we'll go, and if I can get her to 75 percent to 80 percent with the help of doctors and therapists, well then we'll do that. That's where we're going to go."

Therese described the improvements in terms of how well Sami was able to do in school. She started out as the most severe case of autism in her pre-K class, a special class for kids with autism. Three of the parents, like her, were using traditional medicine plus alternative therapies (like her DAN doctor recommended). She said, "All three of those kids who were more on the severe side were, at the end of the year, all at the top of the class. And even the teacher said, 'I don't believe in all this hocus pocus, but I will work with you.'" That teacher worked with the parents to follow dietary restrictions for these kids in the classroom. At the end of the year, Therese told us, the teacher said, "I could get fired for this, for talking to parents about this, but if you would like to share your information, feel free." She was convinced that with efforts like those Sami was following, the ASD symptoms could be reduced.

Therese felt that one of the keys to Sami's improvement was her gut health. She said that early on Sami's digestion was a problem. She was chronically constipated. She was not having normal stools. That was a huge problem, and once they changed her diet, everything else changed.

Therese made sure Sami was on probiotics and all-organic foods. Things got better and better. She described bringing Sami back to her regular pediatrician's office and the new doctor she saw there read her chart and couldn't believe that the original diagnosis was correct.

"We met her and spoke with her and she interacted with Sami," Therese recalled. "The doctor said, 'I'm reading her file and it says she has autism, severe autism, but I'm looking at her and I don't see it. You know, I really don't see it. What is written and what I am seeing, it doesn't match.' She wanted to know everything we had done, and I told her."

By the time Sami was four, Sami's teachers felt she should be "mainstreamed," meaning they recommended she go to regular school. Therese said they gave it a try. Although it was attractive at first, switching back to the regular school turned out to be a disaster. She said Sami appeared to be normal in so many ways. She could have normal conversations and she was intelligent, with lots of creative play. But, what happened is that Therese (and Sami) started to forget about her diet. In the new school, she had no control over what was being served or what Sami ate. Sami started to eat snack foods and carbohydrates: Goldfish, whole wheat bread, high-fructose GM foods that other kids brought to school. Gradually, Sami started to have outbursts and meltdowns and more and more of a difficult time with her mood, throwing tantrums easily. She became sensitive to noise. That went on for a few years and so things gradually got worse and worse.

Therese said she didn't realize how bad it was getting. She kept hoping it was temporary, that it would get a little better, that these were just minor temporary setbacks. But the truth was, there was an overall decline. Therese finally put it all together. "I thought she was cured," Therese said, "so I didn't realize that her care required regular vigilance." When she went back to the pediatrician, Therese said the doctor was amazed at how regressed Sami was. Therese explained how she'd lost track of dietary and supplement protocols, and asked the doctor to run some of the tests she'd had with the DAN doctor. The pediatrician was remarkable, she said; the doctor was totally open to taking Sami back to the DAN doctor. "The pediatrician told us she was convinced that whatever we were doing before was working but that she was hamstrung because she didn't know about any tests for toxic loads or food sensitivities. So she thought the DAN doctor would be more helpful. But he had moved away. So that's when we found Dr. Perro."

When Dr. Perro first met Sami, she realized her case would be challenging. Her mother described how she was throwing tantrums, having meltdowns, screaming, and hitting her. She was chronically constipated again, and could no longer really converse. After getting the full history from Sami's mom, including all of her ups and downs with therapies and symptoms, Dr. Perro crafted a plan to heal Sami's gut. As usual, she changed Sami's diet to get her back on organics and off gluten, soy, and dairy, and used homeopathics. Right away, her mom said, Sami started going to the bathroom again—a sure sign of a more well-functioning gut. Her tantrums, meltdowns, screaming, and hitting subsided. She got back on the vitamin B12 and took probiotics.

Therese described the process of going "back to what we were doing before, to cleaning up her diet, getting her back on the probiotics . . . the whole thing." She said that was how they got Sami back on track. Within a short time, Sami's behavior normalized. As far as Therese was concerned Sami was back to "normal." "She's quirky but not the severe autism we saw," she said. Therese attributed most of the improvement to changes in Sami's diet. She said she should have known this. Sami's father, her husband, was diabetic. Sami's older sister also had problems with digestion. After all this, she had her other daughter do a screen for food sensitivities, and they learned she was sensitive to the same things as Sami: gluten, soy, and dairy. Therese described Sami's sister as seeing huge changes as well. She lost weight and stopped feeling bloated, pudgy, constipated, and mentally foggy. Therese also described her husband's health as improving significantly by following the same diet.

Therese stressed that it wasn't just one thing, but that the food issues were probably the most important part of Sami's recovery. Therese was convinced that it was possible that Sami was predisposed to getting this disorder, probably because she had an inability to detoxify (get rid of toxic metals). As she and her doctors started to remove those things Sami couldn't get rid of on her own, she got better. Therese described Sami's body as being in overload—from the food, the immunizations, all of it. Once they got her detoxed, and once they got the foods she was sensitive to out of her system, she started to come back around.

Was Sami cured of her autism? It's hard to say. But following her mother's assessment, it was clear that many people who met her could no longer tell she was autistic. Therese described what happened last summer at a camp where the family was having a holiday. All the campers were all playing together and one of the other dads came over and said to Therese, "Is your little girl ok? She is wandering off on her own a lot." She told him Sami was diagnosed with autism and the dad said, "Really? I would not have guessed that." According to Therese, "He was just worried she might be having a conflict with the other kids. He was so surprised. He couldn't tell she was autistic."

Dr. Perro recalled the progress with Sami as one of her most treasured moments in her clinical career. When she first met Sami, she was stimming uncontrollably. She couldn't make eye contact. Her speech was monosyllabic and monotone. She was exhibiting profound autism symptoms. She just wasn't "present." Nine months later, when Sami came to her regular appointment, she came into the room and gave her a big hug and said, "Hi, Dr. Perro. How are you?" Dr. Perro and Sami's mom looked at one another and both had tears in their eyes, and smiles of joy on their faces.

Therese wanted to spread the word. She met other parents with kids who had severe autism and she saw them basically "give up" on their kids. "They've taken their doctors' word for it that nothing can be done. But they are wrong," she said. She felt as if just changing the diet made a huge difference for Sami, and that even for kids who were not autistic—kids with ADHD or any mood problems—they could probably also do so much better with the right foods and the right kind of approach.

Leaky Gut, Leaky and Inflamed Brain?

If debates over GMO food science are controversial, then debates over the causes of ASD in America are beyond controversial; they form a virtual snake pit of politics, with hard-hitting campaigns on both sides. Anti-vaxxers (those who are actively campaigning for more research on links between autism and vaccines), as they are called, remain convinced, despite plenty of scientific evidence, that vaccines might be related to the onset of autism symptoms. Pro-vaxxers, on the other side, remain convinced that the overwhelming evidence shows that vaccines are safe and that refusing vaccinations is dangerous.

Many of the debates in the vaccine world replicate those seen in the world of GM food science.[1] Our position is for neither of these polar extremes. Vaccines are vital to individual and public health. We need to keep vaccines in the arsenal for preventing massive and debilitating (as well as deadly) diseases. But we also feel more research is needed to figure out why more and more kids are getting ASD as a diagnosis. This much is clear: The rates of autism are on the rise. The approximation of ASD prevalence is roughly 1 in 68 children today, with a huge preponderance in boys (that is, 1 in 42 for boys, and 1 in 189 for girls).[2] By definition, this has become an epidemic. So, to repeat, we don't advocate against vaccination, but we do think we need more research.

Already, researchers exploring the causes of autism point to the possibility of multifactorial terrain. We know that ASD might be correlated to age of parents at conception or exposure of the mother to toxic chemicals while pregnant. Alcohol and acetaminophen are known potential contributors.[3] Disruptions of the GABA-signaling pathway in the brain (an inhibitory neurotransmitter responsible for reducing excitability) and possibly certain combinations of genes are also associated with autism.[4] There are also calls to explore environmental toxicants in relation to autism.[5] Finally, related to the latter, new research suggests that there are correlations between certain gut bacteria and autism-like behavior based on studies in mice, specifically missing *Lactobacillis reuteri* (one of the key bacteria of the gut microbiome).[6] Mothers with hypothyroidism during pregnancy also have an increased chance of having children on the spectrum.[7] The fact is, we are just beginning to unravel the complexities of the causes of autism and only starting to understand what sorts of therapies help.

There is a small but growing contingent of doctors and scientists who are looking at links between immune system responses and autism.[8] There are proposed pathways between leaky guts and leaky, or inflamed, brains.[9] Could children with an already compromised microbiome or a compromised immune system (which can occur because of a compromised microbiome) be at greater risk for ASD than others? These possibilities need to be explored further.

As more and more kids show up in doctors' offices with cognitive symptoms that warrant a diagnosis of ASD, another perfect storm gathers. Parents often feel quite helpless when presented with this diagnosis in their kids, and this is not surprising. But many physicians also feel quite helpless when presented with cases of ASD. It is virtually impossible to avoid encounters with parents who arrive at the clinic with tears in their eyes and a great deal of anger, sure that their children became autistic from something that happened *to* them. To observe a child who was previously healthy and then presents with an inability to focus, uncontrollable motor symptoms, and regressed behavior is traumatizing for everyone. The patterns are disheartening and frightening, especially when seen over and over again in the clinical setting. Even more dismal is how little there is to offer these parents. Aside from some studies that show that intensive speech, behavioral, and manipulative therapies can provide improvement, there are no real cures for autism in the traditional medical toolbox.

To make matters worse, no two patients who have this diagnosis are exactly alike. This is probably because there are likely to be many different causal pathways and children are affected differently by the same causes. Even diagnostic profiles can look quite different between kids on the spectrum. At best, refining our understanding of the molecular and biochemical mechanisms that seem to be present in ASD has the potential to drive forward strategies for making improvements. Interventions can ameliorate the degree to which these symptoms interfere with normal living. This effort is not just clinical; it is also being done on a societal level as more and more accommodations are created for these children.

Getting Practical with Treatments for Autism Spectrum Disorder

Dr. Perro, like many other integrative practitioners, approaches the situation of ASD with all this in mind. Her focus is on doing things to improve overall cognitive functioning. This means trying to gain a map of the pathophysiology and then systematically trying to correct and repair all of the malfunctioning pathways that are involved. This includes looking at food sensitivities, looking at pathogens in the stool that might produce inflammatory by-products, looking for concomitant infections like yeast, assessing faulty digestion through analysis of protein and fat breakdown products in stool, rebalancing abnormal neurotransmitter levels, repairing problems with methylation and detoxification, and removing heavy metals if they are present in the child (especially lead and mercury, possibly from the mother, environment, and food).

One of the propositions that cases like Sami's point to is that many kids with diagnoses of ASD can get better by therapies that heal the gut. It depends on who the child is, how long they've had the symptoms, and the severity of their symptoms. It also takes a great deal of willpower on the part of the family to make overwhelming changes to get to this end point. But it can happen.

What we know from cases like Sami's is that fixing the gut seems to improve symptoms. So, even if we can't make any firm claims about the causes of autism or its ability to be prevented, it is clear that many kids with autism are able to greatly reduce their symptoms by getting their guts healthy. In fact, it might be possible to minimize them so much that it appears as if they are largely cured, like Sami. ASD in this view starts to look like an affliction that can be reversed, at least in part, for some kids.

This is a tricky issue. Again, there are no magic bullets for most kids with autism, and there are no known cures for some kids born with disabilities that manifest in slow cognitive development from congenital or genetic disorders, or what is referred to as "global delay," as we will see in the next chapter. For many children who have these disorders, the damage to the brain is already done, but we know that the brain is malleable. We would argue that with the right kinds of therapies, many kids with autism or other developmental delay problems should be able to get significantly better. Getting the gut healthy becomes the cornerstone of the therapeutic story.

CHAPTER FIFTEEN

Can Gut Health Improve Other Cognitive Problems?

Once her gut was working, it was as if her brain was waking up.

MOTHER OF KAYLA, a five-year-old patient

Portia had a nearly five-year-old daughter, Kayla, with a developmental disability. Kayla first came to Dr. Perro when she was three years old. According to her mom, Kayla was not diagnosed with autism, even though she had developmental issues that made her look like she was on the spectrum. She was barely sitting even at ten months, and this wasn't normal. She was always constipated, and she had diminished muscle tone. She was not emotional and hardly cried, ever. In fact, the only time she would cry was when she had terrible gas pains. Being constipated for almost a week at a time sometimes meant she would be really gassy and thus in a lot of pain. Her pediatrician had her on MiraLAX every day, which only helped the problem temporarily.

Over the early years, Kayla's parents tried many therapies, including physical, speech, and occupational therapy, with little to no success. Kayla finally got a diagnosis of "global developmental delay," meaning she was not developing normally, but was having delays that stemmed from underlying neurocognitive issues. Portia told us how a stranger overheard her describing Kayla's symptoms to a friend at the grocery store, and how that stranger then came over and told her about how a friend of hers had a child with similar symptoms who had been helped by Dr. Perro. Portia made an appointment with her the next day.

Portia talked about how the positive changes in Kayla's behavior started to show up as soon as they got her off the foods she seemed to be sensitive to. As with most of Dr. Perro's patients, the whole effort included homeopathic remedies, probiotics, a diet of only organic food, and eliminating things that her body had trouble with. It was more than just improved digestion and bowel movements, her mom said. It was like her body was "waking up." Her muscles started to respond. She became more alert, happy, and playful. By four-and-a-half years old, she was still not talking, but she had begun to use simple sign language. She could vocalize to tell people what she wanted and didn't want. Portia described Kayla as needing and seeking a lot of stimulation. She loved going high on the swing and being tossed around with daddy. "She's just really a happy lovely girl in general," her mom said. "She's just not able to form words."

It was clear during the first visit that Kayla was still hyporesponsive. She was the opposite of the type of kid who gets overwhelmed easily by loud noises or big sounds, like Sami in chapter 14. Kayla was also hypotonic, meaning she had low muscle tone. She never tested as autistic, nor did her vision or hearing tests show any abnormalities. Dr. Perro recommended that she undergo a genetic evaluation. Her parents were somewhat hesitant, because there was a high cost involved and there was also some fear of finding out something they didn't want to know. As it turned out, Kayla did have a genetic disorder: a small deletion in one of her chromosomes. Portia thought this might be related to her IVF treatments with her first child. She wondered if she passed on some defect in utero (in gestation) to Kayla.

Portia had formed a theory of what happened to possibly cause Kayla's problems. She told us that she hadn't been able to get pregnant with her son. She tried three rounds of IVF (in vitro fertilization) and it never worked. Then, finally, she got pregnant with her son and it all went well and her son was fine. Her conception of Kayla, however, was a complete surprise. Portia was concerned that all the drugs she had been exposed to (from the IVF) might have been lingering in her system and had an effect on Kayla. She also wondered whether Kayla might have lost oxygen while in utero for a couple of seconds. But the neurologists dismissed her theories. Portia also said that she doubted her daughter's disorder had anything to do with vaccinations. Then there was the chromosomal abnormality.

Portia was not entirely clear what the chromosomal abnormality meant, even though it was clearly involved in Kayla's global developmental delays. But she was also inclined to think Kayla's issues were related to a multiple set of factors. Dr. Perro diagnosed Kayla as a hypomethylator, meaning, like many of the other kids she treated, Kayla was unable to process toxicants well because of a defective MTHFR gene (for methylation). This was confounding her baseline diagnosis that was related to the chromosomal defect.

Despite these issues, Portia thought the most important part of the diagnosis had to do with Kayla's gut function, which only made the delays worse. What Portia was convinced of was that her daughter's gut health and brain health were connected. Portia described how Kayla, from very early on, suffered from gas, bloating, and constipation. Without MiraLAX almost every day of her life, Kayla had suffered. Portia reflected on the fact that the day she changed Kayla's diet, she saw the biggest difference in Kayla.

Following the dietary advice of Dr. Perro, along with homeopathics and supplements, made Kayla not only "regular" but also really happy. All this digestive improvement, Portia said, helped to "wake up her brain." "She's become really active, you can see," she said. "Once her gut was working, it was as if her brain was waking up."

We watched Kayla playing with her mom, trying to get her attention, sitting on her lap and grabbing at her chin when she spoke, laughing, trying to make her mom giggle. She used to just lie there, her mother said. It was as if she had been really distracted or "out of it" and lethargic. But it was amazing now. You could see her connecting. She made eye contact and engaged. She wanted to play. It was really like her brain was just "waking up!"

Dysbiosis and the Afflicted Brain

Understanding the relationship between gut health and brain function means looking not just at microbial communities and missing enzymes and methylators. It means looking at the foods that kids are eating, and tracing from that starting point the ways that different foods impact the body, the microbiome, and the various physiological systems needed for healthy cognitive development. Foods can be beneficial or they can be harmful, and this equation has as much to do with the foods themselves as it does with the body's inherent capacities to digest and use (or eliminate) its various ingredients.

The approach here goes far beyond the simple one-size-fits-all approach to nutrition that has been the cornerstone of dietary advice in medicine for decades. What we are talking about is a much more personalized approach to medicine by way of the gut, and by way of the foods that are put into very specific guts, often in relation to genetic or epigenetic characteristics. If the foods one eats are full of toxic things, they might be hurting more than helping by destroying useful bacteria, making leaks in the epithelium, and slowing digestion (or causing diarrhea, as the case might be). If, further, one does not have the capacity to get rid of these toxic things (because of predispositions such as the methylation defect), these toxicants might end up in the bloodstream, where they travel to the brain and . . . well, who knows?

One way to think of the possibilities here is to note that neither Kayla nor Sami was entirely cured of her disorders, but they both got *significantly* better, so much so that their disorders were no longer recognizably the same. In Sami's case, improvement was so significant that her disability had become invisible to many who met her. In Kayla's case, it was, in her mother's words, "As if she was waking up." Therese was sure that Sami's improvements came from her ability to keep her gut healthy and toxicants out of her body. Similarly, Kayla's mom told us that getting her daughter's diet straightened out was the spark that led to a whole series of bodily awakenings for her. Perhaps, as their guts healed, their brains followed.

One of the explanations that seems plausible in Kayla's case is that her impaired digestion might have been caused by a combination of in-utero exposures and also her own diet that included foods that had a lot of toxicants. These toxicants exacerbated an already poorly functioning digestive tract by creating dysbiosis. When a child has dysbiosis or leaky gut, things get into the bloodstream and are transported to the brain, where, once they pass the blood-brain barrier, they could slow or otherwise impact cognition. We know that neuronal development and functioning require healthy microbial functioning in the gut, but also a healthy nutrient supply. What if you not only don't have the microbes necessary for producing neural proteins, but you also have toxic things entering into the brain by way of the blood? What happens then? We don't know for sure, but we do know that when you get kids' digestion on track and healthy, and get rid of its toxicants, brain function also improves. Perhaps the trick is to give the body the tools and the ecological terrain it needs to heal. This, we argue, begins with organic food.

CHAPTER SIXTEEN

Making Sense of Comorbidities in Children

Here I have a straight A student. She is sort of . . . you know, a driven girl. She knows what she wants to do when she grows up, she has a path that she's on. . . . And all of a sudden she's walking into walls and she's dizzy and her head hurts and she's seeing things. It's as if her brain was shutting down, and now she couldn't even speak anymore.

MOTHER OF STEPHANIE,
a seventeen-year-old patient

Children with multiple chronic physical problems can be incredibly challenging to treat. As we have seen, getting to the root problem can be a long and labored process. Comorbidity, or the presence of one or more additional diseases or concomitant diseases that might occur with the primary disease, is a common problem in kids whose guts are leaky. Disruption of digestion and absorption can impair multiple systems, often all at once. Various disorders can be triggered by a lack of nutrition, including those that affect the brain. As we have discussed, the brain's ability to accomplish sensory processing, from thinking, to feeling, to hearing, to seeing, can be impaired by lack of nutrition and possibly from the presence of toxicants (like pesticides) that find their way into the bloodstream. This can mean not getting critical amino acids or fats that are needed for neural processing, but also, as we have said, it can mean impairment by inflammation from the presence of toxicants in the brain.

In this chapter, we look at the ways in which comorbidities complicate the simple picture of dysbiosis in relation to health. Comorbidities are not just a consequence of intestinal permeability; they can be *a cause* of intestinal permeability, too. If there are missing ingredients in a child's biochemistry (e.g., missing or poorly functioning enzymes), disabilities of key processing functions (e.g., the inability to methylate), or infection by parasites or bacteria (e.g., the bacteria that cause Lyme disease) or from fungal overgrowth, these can also contribute to problems in the gut and, potentially, in the brain.

We have also seen that the therapeutic effort starts with simple changes in the diet: Clear up confounding food intolerances and allergies by clearing out the foods that the body is having a hard time digesting; repopulate the gut with helpful biota that keep the lining of the gut healthy; and enable digestion and absorption to occur normally. This can mean doing something as simple as getting off nonorganic and packaged foods—edible foodlike substances—as with Mike, from chapter 13, the California teen with severe behavioral problems, or Carlos, from chapter 10, who was exposed to pesticides around his home. Sometimes it involves getting rid of foods that appear to be triggers for the immune system, which seems to have been particularly key in Sami's (chapter 14) and Kayla's (chapter 15) cases. Other treatment modalities can get more extensive in complicated patients, such as adding in digestive enzymes to aid patients who might be lacking them for protein and fat breakdown, or adding certain lipids to help repair the nervous system. The treatments are tailored and individualized.

In a fair number of cases, simple dietary remedies can result in vast improvements in children's health. In other cases, however, these improvements do not go far enough. Some symptoms persist, like a lingering cough, recurring headaches, or chronic digestive problems that simply will not clear. In these cases, one has to look beyond diet to other possible augmenting and originating causes. Heading back to the drawing board to rule out or identify other underlying issues can sometimes turn up comorbidities. Let's look at an example of this.

Stephanie's Spiral into Debility, and Her Pathway to Health

Stephanie's story of debility started when she was fourteen years old. She came home from school with severe vertigo and dizziness. Her mother, Stacey, thought it was probably an ear infection. She described the experience of watching Stephanie decline. Stacey was a nurse, so she felt like she could handle it. She kept Stephanie home from school that Friday. But by the following Monday and Tuesday her dizziness was much worse. She started to be so dizzy that she was actually walking into walls. She also started to have a horrible headache on the left side of her head. Stephanie took her to the doctor, who thought she had a severe case of labyrinthitis (inflamed inner ear). He started her on some allergy medicine and scopolamine (for the dizziness). Neither of these helped, and by the end of the week her dizziness was even worse. There was more walking into walls and increased head pain. Stephanie was having to hold onto the walls just to get to the bathroom.

At this point, Stacey was really worried. She still kept Stephanie home from school, and at one point she got a call at her work from Stephanie, who said that she was starting to have episodes where she would lose her vision. Stephanie described these episodes: "I was in the front room watching TV, which is basically all I could do, and I got up to grab an apple or something. I got up not even, not quickly . . . in the second I got up my vision started to get black and fuzzy and it turned straight black, which freaked me out so I grabbed the couch and sat back down really fast. And it lasted like 30 seconds and then stopped." Her vision, she said, came back gradually. It started out kind of gray, and then it started to get wider and more color showed up "sort of like when the sun is starting to rise and you see all the colors around you," she said.

So Stacey took her daughter back to the doctor. At this point Stephanie was also hallucinating; she imagined her mother had a dinosaur on her head. Stacey talked about the panic she was feeling. "Here I have a straight A student. She is sort of . . . you know, a driven girl. She knows what she wants to do when she grows up, she has a path that she's on. . . . And all of a sudden she's walking into walls and she's dizzy and her head hurts and she's seeing things. It's as if her brain was shutting down, and now she couldn't even speak anymore." Stephanie interrupted her mom to tell us that it took her around five minutes just to respond to a yes or no question.

Stacey and Stephanie started a long process of finding a diagnosis. This started with a request for an MRI, which prompted her doctor to ask if she was "faking it." "He thought maybe I was trying to get out of school." He asked if she was doing something in school that was stressing her out. "Didn't she want to go to school?" he asked. This made her angry. Stephanie loved school. She was angry at having to stay home! Finally, her doctor agreed to authorize an MRI, but her report came back normal. At this point the neurologist referred her to a psychiatrist, and they put her on antidepressants. Her dizziness was so bad, she was having to occasionally use a wheelchair.

Stephanie told us that she was also having migraines. And, when her regular doctor looked at the prescription and then heard about the migraines, he told Stephanie and her mom that Stephanie should not be taking that medication. Her physician told them that they were some of the happiest people he knew. Stephanie didn't need antidepressants. But they were still trying to figure out what was going on.

In the meantime, her doctor gave her migraine medicine. She tried Imitrex and that didn't work at all. In all, she tried three or four different medicines. And after several months and some hard-core neural medications that were making her worse, she said "This is not a migraine." Her doctors thought that perhaps if they gave her medicine for her balance they could improve the dizziness and her balance would become better. Instead it made it all worse; everything got worse. At two or three in the morning, Stephanie would start throwing up. So she was getting no sleep and was dizzy all day. This was now a month and a half into it.

Finally, Stephanie was given a CT scan and it showed some cysts in her nasal passages. Stephanie thought these came from the flu shot she was offered at a routine physical exam she had had before she planned to travel with her youth group to an event in Minneapolis (back when she was healthy). The doctor described it as a mist spray, "so she didn't need to get poked." When they got the CT scan back and saw cysts in her sinuses, her doctor said that was an allergic reaction to the FluMist. Taking the FluMist had happened before any of her symptoms appeared. So at that point (after the scan), they felt all of her symptoms were associated with a bad reaction to the FluMist. Three weeks later, they were still saying it was an allergic reaction. They figured that because her sinuses were close enough to her brain, the cysts were putting pressure on her brain. These conditions were causing the headaches and dizziness. A visit to an ENT (ear, nose, and throat doctor) confirmed the cysts in her passages, and that they were very inflamed.

Stacey told us the ENT physician said that Stephanie's passages looked like Swiss cheese and he asked them what she had inhaled. That doctor gave her steroids and suggested that if he could get the inflammation cleared up, the eye symptoms and headaches and everything else would also go away. The steroids did help. They got rid of some symptoms and the nasal passage cysts went away. But all the other symptoms—the headache, the visual problems, the dizziness—that all stayed. Stephanie said, "I was really frustrated. I really wanted a magic pill that would just get rid of all the symptoms."

Instead of things getting better, they got worse. At three months, Stephanie was having so much trouble walking, she was in a wheelchair all the time. Her visual blackouts, blurred vision, and occasional hallucinations persisted. She was always dizzy. She was having lots of muscle and head pain. She had to drop out of school. She couldn't concentrate, could not form sentences. Stacey was getting desperate. The family was really scared. They couldn't figure out what was causing it. Stacey recalled thinking the horrible: that it would have been easier for Stephanie to have something like a brain tumor because then they could start chemo right away or have surgery. She described the horrible feeling, " . . . to imagine that my daughter would be better off with a brain tumor."

It was around this time that Stacey started to take Stephanie to an acupuncturist for pain relief, and that practitioner recommended they try an alternative, and pointed her in Dr. Perro's direction. Stephanie's first visits were an hour and a half, going over her entire history, in detail. Dr. Perro recommended a slew of blood tests, and tests for food allergies and sensitivities. Stacey described feeling relieved initially just because of the attention Dr. Perro paid to the details. The first results that came back suggested that Stephanie had the genes for celiac disease. Dr. Perro also started Stephanie on a series of homeopathic remedies for detoxing. Stephanie described the food therapy as really difficult because her family "basically lived off bread." But it helped her stomach. Stephanie was also started on a series of homeopathic remedies for decreasing inflammation in her stomach and intestines. Those made a big difference, she said. She felt better and her brain began to function better. She thought this was partly because she wasn't dealing with the symptoms from celiac.

About a week later, they got the tests for Lyme disease, one of the tests Dr. Perro ordered, and found out that she tested positive for Lyme disease, as well as *Bartonella*, a coinfection. She didn't know what that was, but her aunt looked it up and told her it was from a tick bite and possibly from a cat scratch. She then remembered she got scratched by a feral cat the year before, just before the symptoms started. A stray cat that was around in her neighborhood came into their house and gave birth to kittens. She told the story of how she was about to put down food for them one time and spooked the cat. "I was separating the kittens from the other animals in the house. We have other dogs. And, well, I guess I spooked her and she scratched my leg." Stephanie thought that might have caused the *Bartonella*. She laughed about the fact that it was hard to know what the real source of all her problems was: "Because you kind of can't prove any of this. Unless you do some giant dissection, which you can't do on a living person," she said. We all laughed. But in fact, all of these problems appeared to be in play and plausible.

Treatment for Stephanie was complicated. To get rid of the chronic infection, Stephanie would have to go on a full course of antibiotics. Because of those, Stephanie described her stomach as being "in bad shape." So, she took tons of supplements and probiotics. And this went on for almost six months. But more of the symptoms were going away. The headache was decreasing. She was also continuing to use various homeopathics as her symptoms improved or changed. The headaches continued to subside. She described them going from a 9 to an 8 to a 7 to a 6 to a 5 at the highest in terms of pain level. She was getting better. The dizziness also decreased. And her visual symptoms, the fuzzy veils (auras) that often accompanied migraines, got a little better. She was still having some of the visual symptoms when we met her. But she pointed out that she was able to walk again. She was out of the wheelchair. She told us she was hoping to be off the walker by her birthday later that month.

After a series of missed diagnoses and many months of struggle, Stephanie and her mother finally felt like they had gotten to the bottom of Stephanie's problems. One could imagine that many of the diagnostic misses and hits in Stephanie's case could have occurred with her regular physician. But Stacey felt that her regular doctors simply weren't equipped to spend the time and do the kinds of diagnostic tests that were finally pursued by Dr. Perro and that ultimately led to her cure.

Lyme disease and its coinfections are controversial, and there are still some doctors who don't understand them well despite a significant amount of literature on the subject and a profound number of patients who suffer with these infections. It can be hard to find a doctor who can deal with these problems, Stacey said. The whole experience of having multiple complex symptoms, of having disorders that were not well understood, and of having doctors who were too quick to dismiss Stephanie's symptoms as psychosomatic, not to mention their quick use of things like the FluMist without explaining its risks, all led her to feel that without the efforts of Dr. Perro, Stephanie would essentially be an invalid.

Stephanie's case reminds us, however, that no matter how much food-related problems are at work in the chronic diseases we see today among kids, most problems are related to, and caused by, complex patterns of comorbidity. When food alone does not fix things, it is important to look beyond at other possibilities.

Thinking about Health from a Systems Perspective

With most chronic, persistent health problems among children, the causes are seldom singular. This makes sense. Bodies are multiplicities; they are not single systems. This is why, although we have focused on food-related ailments, we are not suggesting that food is the only thing that matters when it comes to the health of our kids. Still, it is surprising how often it is absent from our models and our conversations as a core ingredient, or even a starting point, for chronic disorders.

Integrating foods into our models of physiology, pathology, diagnosis, and treatment means thinking about how these basic ingredients of health are impactful in multiple ways. Foods can make us sick, and sometimes our bodies cannot use the foods we are eating to get healthy. In addition to considering foods as both cause and cure for disorders, integrative medicine pays attention to other factors: infections with debilitating bacteria, genetic or epigenetic changes that account for missing elements of methylation, for example, and social situations that can cause stressors that ultimately affect their biochemistry and epigenetics. Chronically ill children require an individualized, multifactorial approach.

Viewing the body as a multiplicity means viewing it as a terrain of synergistic, operational relationships between bacterial (even viral and fungal) and human communities. Embracing these multiplicities means considering multiple entry points for disorders and for treatments. It takes a while to unravel the pathways by which these disorders get set in motion. It also takes time to create new patterns, and to provision the body with the nutrients it needs to function. These efforts, also multiple, at best restore a healthy internal biological and biochemical terrain. They give the organism a chance to, at least, shore itself up against the possibility of living in a toxic world.

If the body is a multiplicity of systems that connect internal to external environments, then how might our efforts to restore health in an internal way reach their limits when the healthy body must return, again and again, to an unhealthy environment? What hopes are there, and what necessity is there, for healing the body in ways that affect the external world? What are the chances that our internal ecologies have anything to teach us about our external ecologies, and, vice versa, how might our insights about external ecosystems help us to heal those that live within us?

CHAPTER SEVENTEEN

Evidence-Based Medicine and Ecosystem Health: Why Not Ecomedicine?

Evidence based medicine (EBM) is the conscientious, explicit, judicious and reasonable use of modern, best evidence in making decisions about the care of individual patients. EBM integrates clinical experience and patient values with the best available research information.

IZET MASIC et al., *Evidence Based Medicine—New Approaches and Challenges*[1]

Over the past half-century of American medicine, the questions of *who* and *what* kinds of evidence to believe when it comes to medical science and clinical care have become more and more difficult to answer. Medicine feels at times up for grabs, with multiple sources of medical knowledge thrown at us and few resources to help us arbitrate these facts. This is true despite the litigious nature of medicine that has made following strict and narrow AMA-established clinical practice guidelines more important than ever.

In fact, many clinicians are feeling pressured, feeling that what they have been taught about chronic disorders might be incomplete, as if there were a crack in the dam. This is partly because medicine today is not simply practiced within clinical spaces; it is practiced through websites that generate public forms of expertise; it is practiced within corporate biotechnology companies and in the ways they fund and prioritize new biomedical research; it is practiced in the halls of schools and playgrounds and on blogs as mothers and caregivers share information about their children's health and healing experiences. The ways in which medical knowledge is produced and shared *have* arguably expanded. Family physicians, drug companies, and scientific researchers are no longer the only sources people listen to when it comes to making decisions about care or treatment options. At the other extreme, medical science moves much faster than the regulatory bodies that govern the standard clinical guidelines.

For these reasons, confusion and frustration can arise for practitioners and patients alike. Standard clinical guidelines sometimes feel out of step with *both* popular opinion and cutting-edge science. Physicians are taught to use evidence-based methods to establish standards of practice, and the public is made to feel comfortable in the belief that their doctors are following these rigorous standards. At the same time, clinicians sometimes feel frustration when they are bound by appointment slots of ten or fifteen minutes with a patient, and when they are faced with patients who come armed with a long list of questions based on what they read online, sometimes even in peer-reviewed scientific articles. What constitutes "good medical care" at a time when patients can sometimes learn as much, if not more, about their ailments from the internet as they can from their doctor?

Frustration in medicine might be, ironically, one of the logical outcomes of efforts to make medicine more scientific, not just because patients can read the science themselves. As guidelines for practicing medicine become increasingly driven by evidence-based science, efforts that don't conform to these guidelines are increasingly scrutinized, even when past successes in clinical care and outcomes for these procedures are well known. Evidence-based medicine has perhaps unwittingly produced a sense that clinical practices are becoming unmoored from their solid scientific foundations as more and more care practices are arbitrated by clinicians and patients alike, and the bar for achieving "good scientific evidence" is raised higher and higher.

One can see this vividly in the debates over the utility of the case study. Clinicians who have for a century or more relied on case studies that attest to success (both in their own practices and in peer-reviewed medical journals) are now told that case studies are unreliable in the face of randomized controlled trial forms of evidence. Case studies are now called "anecdotal" as forms of evidence, and they are made to seem less valid than evidence produced in experimental randomized controlled trial studies. Along with this (and perhaps in part because of this), patients seem increasingly inclined to follow personal experiences with success and evidence they glean from the scientific literature on their own. Clinicians often feel caught between a rock and a hard place when faced with these behaviors and the new hierarchies of evidentiary validity. Do they follow the evidence-based guidelines or do they follow what their clinical experience has shown them, even when there is not a substantial evidence base to support it? All of this leads to a good deal of exasperation in the medical world, not only among patients but also among physicians. Nowhere is this more problematic than in the case of chronic disorders.

Indeed, while modern medicine offers extraordinary acute interventions that are more precise, more complex, and, in most cases, more effective than ever before, it also continues to struggle with effective diagnosis and treatment for many chronic debilitating health conditions. We can transplant kidneys and hearts, but we have trouble treating chronic allergies, autoimmune disorders, and many mental health problems. In some ways, chronic conditions define the limits of modern medicine; ailments become chronic when they are not cured. Increasingly, clinicians are seeing patients who are given more and more drugs and yet there are as yet no cures for their underlying problems. No matter how scientifically valid the efforts of clinical care might be, if the patient is not healed, the search for a cure will go on, particularly when the patient is a child.

In this book, we have pointed to the fact that many theories of food-related health and healing are not found in established AMA clinical guidelines because there is not yet a sufficient evidence base established by randomized, controlled clinical studies that shows simple changes in diet can ameliorate many of these chronic problems in part or *in toto*. Dr. Perro joins many forward-thinking clinicians who are personally convinced of these new approaches on the basis of studies that have been done on animals or on the basis of the evidence from genetic, molecular, and biochemical in vitro analyses of these things. There is, after all, a growing literature that establishes links between pesticides, genetic modifications, and other toxicants and poor health in animals, as well as biochemical studies of the properties of these chemicals. Still, this does not mean the information they find in the annals of bioscience journals have found their way into medical journals and standard clinical practice guidelines. This is so important, and it is the link that we are trying to call attention to in this book.

There are several reasons for the gap that currently exists between clinical guidelines and new scientific information. First, the bar for doing clinical trials research that can change AMA clinical guidelines is very high, and for a good reason. Doing scientifically valid randomized controlled studies of medical therapies takes significant time, large numbers of human subjects, and heaps of money. Even using other kinds of evidence—epidemiological studies, clinical case studies, or case-controlled studies—also takes a great amount of all three. Because the bar is so high, the standards rather narrow, and the cost so prohibitive, clinical guidelines are generally conservative and slow to change. In addition to this, much of the funding for such studies comes from the industries that medicine has partnered with over the years—including the pharmaceutical and biotechnology industries. Some question the AMA's inherent bias toward industry-funded approaches to care. This same bias is found in the research on food and food production technologies in relation to health. Many of the studies done by biomedical industries are oriented only toward those interventions, the pharmaceuticals and technologies that they are selling (we looked at some of these trends in chapter 3).

The conspiracy of factors in this situation leads to monopolies on knowledge production that leave suspicious and inquisitive clinicians to fend for themselves in trying to find solutions that are not tied to these industries. This is even truer for those trying to scrutinize impacts of things like the food technologies we use today. What goes on in the laboratories of agricultural science is seldom considered by doctors, let alone translated into treatment programs for patients, particularly for children. In fact, the clinical guidelines are set by agencies that are worlds apart from the research institutes working on GM foods and, as we have seen, if these agencies rely on reports from the FDA and EPA alone, they will not be worried about the relationships between GM foods (and their pesticides) and health. The question of how safe agrochemically produced and readily available supermarket foods are is simply not part of the clinical practice repertoire.

Moving Beyond "Pill for Ill" Medicine: Focusing on Food Health

Jonathan Latham, executive director of the Bioscience Resource Project, notes that just as our foods have become genetically engineered, we have been engineered by culture to believe that food is not important to health.[2] Ironic as this sounds, it is largely true. When we are sick, clinicians are likely to run a series of lab tests that are designed not to uncover root causes but to offer symptomatic relief through pharmaceuticals. We try to figure out what gene, what biochemical malfunction or pathogen has caused the ailment rather than considering that food has anything to do with it. (Of course, many tests are needed to find out what our bodies *are doing* when exposed to different foods, too.) Many of the stories of frustrated patients in this book attest to the reluctance among most clinicians to consider that food could be a root cause of their disorders. Most clinicians are trained to turn first to their pharmaceutical arsenal to make their patients better, or to at least make them feel better, because this is how they were trained and because these drugs often work well, up to a point. (It's what Dr. Perro called "Pill for Ill" medicine in chapter 2.) Thinking beyond the box of pharmaceutical solutions is difficult, if only because we have so many pharmaceuticals to choose from for virtually any and all symptoms, not to mention that patients also want quick fixes and magic bullet solutions even, or sometimes especially, when a disease is chronic.

We cannot entirely abandon our reliance on pharmaceuticals. In fact, many food-focused doctors also rely on a bevy of pharmacological products or technologies. Indeed, many integrative therapies rely on products that are industrially produced, including supplements, vitamins, remedies, and other products, even if they argue that these products are "natural." We also can be sure that some of the research on the microbiome is likely to push discovery of even more pharmaceuticals for repairing the gut, rectifying the microbiome, or reducing the body's natural response to problematic foods (much as we see in therapeutic drugs for those with food intolerances). In fact, some large pharmaceutical companies are in the business of producing green pharmacy products that are used in integrative medicine, so the lines between pharmaceutical versus food solutions are blurring. We can't be too black and white here; most therapies will involve both efforts. At the same time, it would be a mistake to assume that pharmaceuticals could replace food as a starting point for health and disease, diagnosis and treatment. And, in the end, our pharmaceutical companies are far more likely to produce drugs and high-tech solutions to our health problems than they are to focus on cleaning up our food supply.

We would argue that in order to do the kind of clinical care that advances the proposition that food is integral to health, physicians will have to think beyond the pill. We all need to think about how preventing diseases before they start means looking at more basic things like the food we eat, the quality of its nutritional composition, and the possibility that it is laden with toxicants.

What we are saying here is that we need a type of medicine that understands how patients are part of a medico-environmental ecosystem, what we call *ecomedicine*. Considering food-related causes of ill health means thinking beyond the normal list of diseases that students are currently taught in medical school and also beyond the normal list of drug therapies that are available for these diseases. In the ecomedicine ecosystem, foods, bodily health, and even political activism all matter in the effort to create an approach in which ill health and its causes can be assessed and understood. In this ecosystem, health can be sought and achieved only if the food ecosystem is itself healthy. In this ecosystem, the notion of cleaning up our food supply seems like an obvious starting place. In this sense it is worth thinking a little more about how healthy our food ecosystem is, *or is not*.

Heathy Soil, Plants, and People: We Are All Part of the Same Ecosystem

While many agrochemical industry advocates and supporters continue to applaud the extraordinary transformations of our food supply systems by noting that food is now more available, affordable, safe from pests and weeds, and nutritious, we have shown that there is ample evidence to the contrary. Against the intransigent supporters of our agroindustrial empire, we argue that industrialized food production has depleted the environments where it is used, requires huge supplements of chemically rich products to survive, has compromised the nutritional value of these foods, has created huge dependencies of farmers on subsidies, has rendered our agricultural system vulnerable, is pathologic to human health, and is basically at a dead end.

Andrew Kimbrell, from the Center for Food Safety, says that industrial agriculture is a *zombie paradigm*.[3] We have so depleted the environment of its health that, in order to keep it alive, we now have to use technologies and chemicals in increasing amounts every year just to keep ahead of the wreckage. It is alive, but it is as if dead. From the soil and its living inhabitants that are wiped out by pesticides to the declining ecosystem health of water, we now need to use supplemental techniques (with chemicals, nutrients, and microbes) to grow our food. We are witnessing a food production system that is chronically on life support.

If nothing else, our hope is that in reading this book you have been convinced to take a second look at the problems of the rise of toxicants in our environment from industrialized forms of food production and the rise in chronic, persistent, hard-to-diagnose health problems in our children. We have also argued that integrative food-focused medicine is at the receiving end of the spoils of this agroindustrial system, seeing kids with chronic disorders who have struggled to find effective clinical care. As a consequence of having worked our way through these problems—this perfect storm of a medical system that fails to take food seriously, a food industry that allows us to poison our foods, and a scientific community that is only beginning to understand how our bodies work as multispecies ecosystems—we hope that many will feel better equipped to respond to, or at least to navigate through, the often frustrating world of chronic ailments in new ways. At a minimum, we hope that you are provoked to think about the need for current clinical practice guidelines to deal more directly with food-related health problems. How might we move the dial toward food-focused medicine so that it would be less resistant to exploring the connections between *how we grow our food* and *how we grow our health*?

Rethinking Our Industrial Food and Pharmaceutical Systems Together

What can be done to prevent an eye roll at the mere mention of critiques of GM foods? To begin with, *we need to move beyond the simple argument that we should not be tampering with nature.* Humans have since the dawn of time been engaged with a process of taming and tampering with nature in order to feed themselves. The mere notion of agriculture is, by definition, an act aimed at controlling and modifying nature. What we are concerned with, and what the GM-food debate should focus on, is how the use of genetic technologies and pesticides to grow our foods has resulted in fundamental changes to the foods themselves, and consequently to those of us who eat them. The presumption underlying this critique is that in order to have a safe food supply, we must move beyond the linear battle between the good (foods) and evil (threats to food supply) and instead think about ecosystem survival.

Our food production model is like our outdated medical model: Crops need to be protected from invasive pests and competitors by developing better weapons (read: chemicals or technologies) to kill them (even turning our foods into such weapons). We need to come up with some new paradigms. Just as the pharmaceutical companies wrested control over diagnosis and treatment, so, too, have the technology and chemical agricultural industries wrested control over our food production systems. The pharmaceutical companies' hold over medicine has pushed medicine inexorably in the direction of drugs. Similarly, agricultural industries have pushed food production more and more toward solving all their problems by using stronger and more dangerous chemicals and technological fixes. Just as pharmaceutical industries have performed miracles in pharmaceutical medicine while also creating eddies of chronicity for which there are few good miracle drugs, agrochemical industries have been quite profitable in solving our food production problems in this way. But the lion's share of profits has gone to companies, while consumers and farmers have had to pay the high price of this war. The agrochemical industries have also created huge eddies of chemical waste that now finds its way into the bodies of our children. The war on food pests, like the war on ill health, has had huge spoils, in both the positive financial sense but also in the negative human sense. On this note, the winning bid by Bayer Pharmaceuticals to purchase Monsanto Corporation in late 2016 offers much to ponder, especially about the potential for doubling down on the profits from agrochemicals that, ironically, generate greater and greater need for pharmaceutical therapies because of the chronic diseases these agrochemicals cause.

When those who recommend returning to effective, nontechnology-based solutions to our current health crises are called "antiscience," we say: Look at the evidence. The evidence suggests that the use of organic nonindustrial forms of food production is not necessarily antiscience, nor is it in any sense going backward from science. It is the logical, and rational, path forward. Growing our food in the industrial and chemically dependent, genetically modified ways that we have so far is not good for our health. In order to get healthy, we have to rethink and redo the ways we eat and produce food.

We are not the first to make this case and we are in good company: Rachel Carson, Frances Moore Lappé, Michael Pollan, Vandana Shiva, Robert F. Kennedy, Jr., Winona LaDuke, and a host of others have made compelling cases for this necessary revolution in our food production systems (some who are more strident than others). And this is before we get to more recent and powerful cases that are made by authors like Daphne Miller, Stacy Malkan, Caitlin Shetterly, Jeffrey Smith, and Robyn O'Brien (among others) whose books trace the important links between unhealthy (read: contaminated) GM food and unhealthy people, not to mention well-known committed activists like Zen Honeycutt (Moms Across America) and Pamm Larry (GMO Free

USA). Our message, like theirs, is that the strongest case we can make for needed changes is right in our own sick children.

So many ill children reveal the ways we have outgrown our medical model and our predominant food production systems. The problems our kids suffer from most persistently today are complex, arising from a multisystem dysfunctional biological catastrophe, particularly in relation to immunity, autoimmunity, and the health sequelae that arise from these problems. These diseases suggest a body that is both confused and collapsing under the pressure of so many toxic exposures. If we are looking for evidence that our food systems have failed us, we should pay attention to these children. We have a generation of children whose chronic illnesses do not resemble those of the previous generations. Our kids are sicker than their parents, and arguably sicker than their parents were when they were children, regardless of our agricultural and pharmaceutical "advances." Clinical evidence indicates that we are doing something wrong. Quite possibly what we are doing wrong today started with the changes to our food production that began just before most of these kids were born. The vital question is: How do we get out of this mess?

These problems require systemic change—changes throughout all of the body's biological systems, our medical understanding and health systems, and our food production systems simultaneously. What we are proposing is an approach that nurtures food ecosystems that simultaneously nurture healthy environments and healthy bodies. Whether we conceptualize this at the level of the soils and their multiple living species that are required to stay healthy, or at the level of the gut microbiome that also needs a plethora of healthy species to survive, the model is one that looks for symbiotic modes of engagement—where mutual sustainability is possible. Food becomes a message and messenger, diplomat and language, decoder and purveyor of options derived from the relationships outside and inside the body. We are proposing, or reinforcing for some, the idea that the limiting factor in health is our food environment; our internal ecosystems are only going to be as healthy as our external environmental ecosystems. The provision of healthy, nutritious, and nontoxic food is in this sense a public health concern.

If we took seriously the ecological proposition that the human body is a living microcosm dependent upon the multiplicity of organisms that coinhabit the world, would this approach enable us to look for systemic disruptions in living systems that show up inside the body as inner symptoms of outer imbalances that could be repaired? What kinds of tools might we need to repair these symbiotic relationships? What role might food play in finding this dynamic balance? If this were common knowledge among consumers, would the profit industries that have garnered outsized power with regulatory and scientific agencies be amenable to these changes, just as farmers are starting to realize that organic growing might actually increase their profits? What would it mean to restructure our approaches to food, health, and healing in ways that altered the focus of the large agrochemical industries and their scientific infrastructures that have for so many years convinced us that their current approach to food production is the only viable way to feed the masses in our modern world?

Seeing the larger profit margins from organics, even conventional growers are starting to figure out how to convert to organics, based on economic viability. But this, too, is a problem. Organic food supply chains should not be available only to the rich and well located. They should be available to everyone. Government subsidies of organic farmers is an easy solution to this problem, just as conventionally grown foods are subsidized presently with tax dollars.

How do we get there? We believe we need medical science to throw its weight in this direction, to make the connections between the threatened health of our future generations and the ways we are provisioning them with food. What is missing is consensus from science and medicine that states, boldly and unequivocally, that organic food is not only better for health but also imperative to a healthy food production system. There are a few established medical organizations that have made public statements about this. The American Academy of Environmental Medicine, for instance, has published a position statement against consumption of GM foods on the grounds that their safety has yet to be proven, and there is controversial evidence that they might be harmful.[4] But this is not enough.

If the organic farming community is on board with this idea (and has in fact been actively resisting agrochemical companies for a long time), and if the public is largely on board (they want, and when possible they buy, organic foods, in particular foods that are labeled non-GMO), then what is the holdup? Taking the science seriously. That is why we wrote this book.

If our present medical model works against the type of healthy paradigm switches we are talking about, we need to change that model. Already, integrative approaches are being incorporated into the primary care system in many places. But even food-focused clinicians can do only so much. The burden of care for sick kids continues to fall on the patients' parents, often moms, who in turn become the most important adversary and advocate in this battle to improve medicine and clean up our food supply. It is to these women we now turn in our final chapter.

CHAPTER EIGHTEEN

Warrior Moms: The Call to Action

What kind of future do we want to hand down to our kids?

Activist, Friends of the Earth

One of the more compelling reasons for writing this book comes from our overwhelming sense that we need to support the growing number of families, and particularly the mothers, of children with chronic debilitating and pernicious disorders who are already fighting the good fight for healthy foods. These women describe themselves as driven, against all obstacles, to get their kids healthy. Their stalwart efforts are not just against the symptoms that ravage their kids' bodies and minds, that derail them from school, that leave them miserable on a daily basis. Their effort is toward something much larger. In many ways, they want to change the world.

This won't be, and has not been, easy. Moms who find their way to food-focused solutions for their children's ailments are frequently met with opposition on multiple fronts. Sometimes opposition comes from their regular doctors and caregivers who, at best, disregard their therapeutic choices or, at worst, actively petition against them. Though by far the most frustrating source of opposition, these moms say, is from within their own families and communities. Grandparents who feel these mothers are being overprotective. Husbands who think that eliminating foods or eating only organic foods is simply ridiculous and unnecessarily costly. Friends, teachers, and even colleagues who discreetly criticize these moms for going to such lengths to control what their kids eat. . . . There are moments when a mother (or primary caregiver) has to summon up all her strength and push back against the mainstream.

We all know mothers who fit this description. The moms who package special snacks for their kids' after-school playdates and who insist on teachers monitoring lunchtime to make sure their children are not sharing the risky foods of classmates. We all know the grandparents, aunts and uncles, and even spouses who use every opportunity to slip that favorite ice cream, macaroni and cheese, or glazed donut into the mouths of these kids who they think are otherwise being denied these so-called pleasures. We all know the sentiments that lie just below the surface about these moms, the not-so-hidden cynicism that these moms are "food crazy," "neurotic," and "helicopter moms." Criticism mounts that their kids' problems probably have more to do with their mothers' obsessions than with these kids' toxic predicaments from the foods they are eating. The fact that these kids often have siblings who are perfectly healthy only adds to these sentiments. We see this sort of cynicism even when the kids' ailments are well known, visible, and obviously painful for the children. Helen's story about her daughter, Sylvie, offers a good example of this. We turn to her story now, as a final clinical case study, to remind others who have been in this situation that they are not alone.

Helen's Commitment to Her Daughter's Health

Sylvie's mother, Helen, described what she thought caused Sylvie's severe eczema. It started very early on, Helen said. She started getting rough and red patches at about five weeks old. She said she read about it and consulted doctors, who told her it was probably related to hormones. The doctors told her that Sylvie's body was going through withdrawal from hormones. The doctors told her it would go away, but to Helen, it was more than a mild case of eczema that would clear up on its own. She herself had suffered from eczema most of her life, but her daughter was only a few weeks old. It was alarming. She felt like it was finally time to figure out what was really causing it, even if it was hormones, or what could fix it. In her terms, she wanted to "get to the bottom of it."

Helen talked about not wanting her daughter to have to go through what she went through as a child. She had eczema behind her knees and recalled walking with a sweatshirt to cover that area because it was so inflamed and very red and embarrassing. Of course, she used steroidal creams when she had flare-ups, but she was loathe to give them to her baby. So she started Sylvie on special nonsteroidal creams, hoping that would help.

When Sylvie was about five months, Helen was also seeking a remedy for her own poor health. In addition to recurring eczema, she also had recurring diarrhea. She found an integrative doctor who ran a number of tests and told her that she had huge magnesium deficiencies as well as elevated metals. He got her started on probiotics and detoxing supplements such as chlorella. This explained, she said, why her skin was always so inflamed. This was her weakest link—her gut.

Helen figured that since she was still breastfeeding, clearing up her issues would also help her daughter. In fact, she noticed that when her own symptoms would flare up, so would Sylvie's.

When Helen finally found Dr. Perro, Sylvie was about fifteen months old. Right away, Dr. Perro got Sylvie off gluten and dairy and then started to work on repairing her gut with a combination of homeopathics and probiotics. This helped a lot, Helen said, and it was amazing to see how much more clear Sylvie's skin was. But the eczema didn't go away completely. She would still have flare-ups periodically. They were more subtle than before, but they still recurred. When they moved to a new home, Sylvie suddenly got much worse, with symptoms so bad that her teachers suggested that she stay home from preschool.

Helen described her difficult situation as one in which even her parents started to question her choice of using integrative medicine instead of simply bathing Sylvie in steroid creams. Her biggest challenge, she said, was dealing with the constant pushback and skepticism from her physician father and from Sylvie's friends' parents. "They just don't get it," she said, "even though they can see the results [from her strict dietary care for Sylvie]." She felt isolated a lot of the time. Playdates, for instance, took a huge amount of planning: Helen had to make sure that the family where Sylvie was going was not going to give Sylvie foods that would make her sick, or Helen just orchestrated her playdates at her home. She mostly had to manage all of this on her own, because there weren't many other moms who sympathized with the issues or whose kids had the same kinds of problems.

Helen described her natural tendency to steer preschool friendships toward other kids whose parents were also trying to be careful about food. She had a good sense that given how many foods Sylvie was exposed to that were dangerous for Sylvie, she *had to be* somewhat obsessive. Helen didn't have a choice. These foods are not just going to disappear from the food landscape, she said. Thankfully, Dr. Perro and Helen discovered that with additional vitamins and minerals, Sylvie could actually stabilize her reactions to some of these exposures, which made life much easier for both Helen and Sylvie. But still, keeping Sylvie safe from foods that would undermine her gut health was a continuous effort that took constant vigilance and, in Helen's view, a "warrior-like" commitment.

In the end, Dr. Perro found out that Sylvie, like many of her patients, had a methylation deficiency. Helen also got tested and learned she, too, had the deficiency. Helen explained how the deficiency alone was not a problem, but if you are exposed to lots of toxicants, then the load of what you need to detoxify goes up. She described how you could modulate the symptoms partly by being careful with food. "When you're exposed to GM foods and pesticides or what have you, that's huge." Sylvie's body, she said, just wasn't able to get rid of those poisons. "If you're someone like my husband, who doesn't have a problem, it's fortunate to not have to worry about it. But she did [have to worry]."

Helen supplemented Sylvie's diet with methyl folate, vitamin B6, and methyl B12, as well as minerals, particularly increased doses of zinc because she showed a deficiency of that mineral. In addition, she was treated with an omega three from pasteurized cod liver oil and continued with probiotics with large amounts of beneficial bacteria. Dr. Perro added glycine, which is an amino acid that helps with detoxification. Within a couple of months, Sylvie's skin got significantly better. The difference, Helen said, was *huge*.

Helen described remembering painfully watching her daughter sit and scratch and scratch until her poor limbs were swollen and bleeding.

These days, she said, since using the treatments Dr. Perro gave Sylvie, she was eczema-free most of the time. Her flare-ups were rare, but as far as she could tell, they were definitely related to food. Still, Helen had to contend with the constant threat that Sylvie would get offered scones (from grandma and grandpa) or a piece of pizza (from friends at school) and the symptoms would return. It was frustrating to have these setbacks, even though her mother tried so hard to keep Sylvie on a strict diet.

Committing to Change on an Individual and Societal Level

Many of the mothers who have figured out that food is the key to their children's health have also figured out that this effort must go beyond their homes and their neighborhoods. They know that even undertaking the simple act of making good food choices in grocery stores requires having the option to buy good foods in those stores in the first place. These mothers have taken on political efforts to quite literally change the food landscape in the United States, at least, if not the world. For many, especially those whose children are very young, the effort takes place on the home front, in schools, and in local communities. For others, the battle carries them to much larger theaters of debate. We call these moms "warrior moms"; they are leading us in the movement to eliminate our chronic exposures and ensure the health of our future generations.

These mothers are working to provision communities with organic foods in places where they might not yet be available. They advocate for labeling of GMOs in the foods that are available and for eradicating pesticide spraying on farms and local parks. They call for funding independent research that will explore how the processes we use to grow our food matter in life and death sorts of ways. We have listed some of the organizations they are working with in the Resources section at the end of this book. There are hundreds of small, locally active, and successful nongovernmental, grassroots groups that are doing amazing work (and not all were started by mothers). Frequently, these women have learned from their own very personal experiences with their sick children that the problems their kids face are much larger than themselves and their own kids. They are problems that must be tackled at a much higher level than just their own food choices.

Like the moms who are chastised by friends and family behind their backs in the PTA meetings and on the playgrounds for being overprotective of their children's diets, activist moms are also harassed. Internet trolls call them "sancti-mommies"—an insult meant to suggest women who act sanctimonious about their health and their food. Critics dismiss them as not credible, self-promoting, and naïve.

These trolls couldn't be more wrong. These moms have often learned the hard way, because of their experiences with their own children, that some things have to be fought for, against many odds. We think these moms are absolutely worth listening to. One of the most important tenets of good pediatric care taught to interns and residents in the United States is: *Listen to the parents!* We believe these parents, and particularly these moms, are our frontline warriors in the movement to get our kids—*all kids*—healthy by making our food safe. We need to take their stories and their activism seriously. In solidarity with these moms, we need to rethink our models of food production from the inside out, just as we need to heal the bodies of our children from the inside out. The healthy transitions we need to make within our microbiome must extend to changes in the outside world. Clinicians need to be at the front of this battle alongside the moms, the activists, and the leading-edge scientists who are already showing us the way to a healthier future.

What if pediatricians and the larger medical community were to recognize what these moms have already discovered? What would it take to get these insights, and the growing evidence base of these links, into standard clinical guidelines for pediatric care? What if health professionals and their patients were to unite behind the common cause of providing food security and food safety by supporting more funding for research and more careful regulation? This call to action will require many communities to step up and come forward: the scientists, the politicians, the educators, and the farmers. Together these groups might unify, bridge their unique disciplines, and provide the impetus for change.

ACKNOWLEDGMENTS

We are deeply grateful to the mothers, fathers, and children who shared their stories for this book. We are also grateful to many friends and colleagues who read drafts or portions of drafts of the book, including Debbie Friedman, Michael Antoniou, Claire Robinson, Myrto Ashe, Sharon Kaufman, Arianna Van Meurs, Sienna Craig, Elsie Kelly, Lydia Norby-Adams, Lindsay Berkowitz, Dana Greenfield, and Howard Vlieger. We deeply appreciate the research assistance provided by Sayles Day, whose insights from literature on the microbiome are found throughout this book. We appreciate the publishing advice from Beth Greer and Randy Peyser. We appreciate the counsel and pathbreaking work of colleagues at UCSF, Stanton Glantz, Tracey Woodruff, and Patrice Sutton and the team at the Environmental Health Institute. Our acknowledgment of these persons does not imply their endorsement for any of the views presented here. We could not have completed this book without the generous and painstaking help of Claire Robinson and Michael Antoniou, whose work in this field, each in his and her own way, is exemplary, guided by ethics, integrity, and intellectual commitment. Our publishing team at Chelsea Green has been superb, as has been our agent, Sharon Bowers.

In the larger pool of persons who have influenced this work, we want to thank Mark Squire and Good Earth Natural Foods for supporting the organic movement and enabling us to eat healthy foods while we wrote the book. We acknowledge and appreciate the fruitful conversations and insights generated by the group at GMO Science, as well as several workshops they organized, the crew at Paicines Ranch, and the event at the home of John and Betty Gaye Potter.

Michelle thanks her family (Rich, Jesse, and Anji), who have sat through many years of talks and lectures, friends (Sandy Gartzman, who has listened to the GM story on many a long hike), and her patients for their patience and for being a continuing source of inspiration in what is often uncharted territory. She extends a heartfelt thank you to Dr. Arpad Pusztai for his groundbreaking work, and to Jeffrey Smith whose book *Seeds of Deception* first showed her the light and got her started on the path of GM food research and health. And, finally, she thanks Vincanne for her willingness to take on this project, as well as her exceptional academic rigor, curiosity, and talent at turning this complex topic into digestible bites.

Vincanne thanks her husband, John Norby, for his persistent, loving, and generous engagement as the partner of an academic. She also thanks her children, family and friends, and students (especially Raphael Frankfurter and Caroline Hodge for a test round of the material with medical students), as well as her institution (UCSF) for being the sort of place that embraces critical research and investigation. She thanks Stacy Leigh Pigg and the audience at Simon Fraser University for feedback on a short version of a piece of the book. She thanks Michelle for staying in the courageous fight to help our kids, for venturing into the lesser-known but critical new pathways being forged in the integrative health world, and for getting her involved in this important field of study and work.

Resources

BOOKS, FILMS, AND ORGANIZATIONS CONCERNED WITH GM FOODS OR RISING CHRONIC DISEASE

Books

Achieving Victory over a Toxic World: An Inspirational Story That Will Lead You to Eye-Opening Revelations about the Impact the Environment Has on Your Health, by Mark A. Schauss (AuthorHouse, 2008)

The Autism Revolution: Whole-Body Strategies for Making Life All It Can Be, by Martha Herbert, MD, with Karen Weintraub (Ballantine Books, 2013)

Brain Maker: The Power of Gut Microbes to Heal and Protect Your Brain for Life, by David Perlmutter, MD, with Kristin Loberg (Hatchette Digital, 2015)

The Disease Delusion: Conquering the Causes of Chronic Illness for a Healthier, Longer, and Happier Life, by Jeffrey S. Bland, PhD (Harper Wave, 2014)

Grain Brain: The Surprising Truth about Wheat, Carbs, and Sugar—Your Brain's Silent Killers, by David Perlmutter, MD, with Kristin Loberg (Little, Brown and Company, 2013)

Gut and Psychology Syndrome: Natural Treatment for Autism, Dyspraxia, A.D.D., Dyslexia, A.D.H.D., Depression, Schizophrenia, by Natasha Campbell McBride, MD (Medinform Publishing, 2010)

Seeds of Deception: Exposing Industry and Government Lies about the Safety of the Genetically Engineered Foods You're Eating, by Jeffrey Smith (Yes! Books, 2003)

Super Natural Home: Improve Your Health, Home, and Planet—One Room at a Time, by Beth Greer (Rodale Books, 2009)

Wheat Belly: Lose the Wheat, Lose the Weight, and Find Your Path Back to Health, by William Davis, MD (Rodale Books, 2014)

Why Can't I Get Better? Solving the Mystery of Lyme and Chronic Disease, by Richard Horowitz, MD (St. Martin's Press, 2013)

The World According to Monsanto, by Marie-Monique Robin (The New Press, 2010)

Movies

Genetic Roulette: The Gamble of Our Lives, by Jeffrey Smith, Institute for Responsible Technology, 2012, http://geneticroulettemovie.com (see also the book of the same name)

Scientists under Attack: Genetic Engineering in the Magnetic Field of Money, by Bertram Verhaag, Denkmal Films, 2010, http://responsibletechnology.org/resources/scientists-under-attack/

Secret Ingredients, by Jeffrey Smith and Amy Hart, Institute for Responsible Technology, expected release date January 2018, trailer available at: https://www.youtube.com/watch?v=CnXG3-Vt2Ps

Seed: The Untold Story, by Taggart Siegel and John Betz, Collective Eye Films, 2017, http://www.seedthemovie.com

The World According to Monsanto, by Marie-Monique Robin, 2015, https://www.youtube.com/watch?v=zfOSFaaLx_o (see also the book of the same name)

Websites

Allergy Kids Foundation https://robynobrien.com/allergy-kids-foundation
Center for Food Safety http://www.centerforfoodsafety.org
The Conscious Kitchen http://www.consciouskitchen.org
Food and Water Watch http://www.foodandwaterwatch.org
Friends of the Earth http://www.foe.org
GMO Free California http://www.gmofreeca.org/
GMO Science http://www.gmoscience.org
GM Watch http://www.gmwatch.org
Good Earth Natural Foods http://www.genatural.com
Institute for Responsible Technology http://responsibletechnology.org
Just Label It http://www.justlabelit.org
Made Safe http://www.madesafe.org
Moms Across America http://www.momsacrossamerica.com
Moms Advocating Sustainability http://www.momsadvocatingsustainability.org
Non-GMO Project http://www.nongmoproject.org
Organic Consumers Association http://www.organicconsumers.org
Pesticide Action Network http://www.panna.org
US Right to Know https://usrtk.org

NOTES

Introduction

1. During the twentieth century, infant mortality in America was reduced by 90 percent (from roughly 100 to roughly 8 per 1,000 live births). Public health, nutrition, and medical efforts eliminated most causes of childhood mortality, setting an example for the rest of the world. "Achievements in Public Health, 1900–1999: Healthier Mothers and Babies," Centers for Disease Control and Prevention, MMWR Weekly 48, no. 38 (October 1, 1999): 849–58, https://www.cdc.gov/mmwr/preview/mmwrhtml/mm4838a2.htm.
2. Specifically, this rate is for 1997 to 2011. "Food Allergy Facts and Statistics for the U.S," Food Allergy Research and Education, accessed March 3, 2016, https://www.foodallergy.org/file/Final-FARE-Food-Allergy-Facts-Statistics.pdf.
3. Ronit Herzog and Susanna Cunningham-Rundles, "Pediatric Asthma: Natural History, Assessment and Treatment," Mount Sinai Journal of Medicine 78, no. 5 (September/October 2011): 645–60, doi:10.1002/msj.20285; "Asthma in the US: Growing Every Year," Centers for Disease Control and Prevention, posted May 2011, accessed July 7, 2016, http://www.cdc.gov/vitalsigns/asthma; "National Center for Health Statistics: Asthma," Centers for Disease Control and Prevention, accessed July 7, 2016, http://www.cdc.gov/nchs/fastats/asthma.htm; Lara J. Akinbami, "The State of Childhood Asthma, United States, 1980–2005," Advance Data from Vital and Health Statistics 381 (revised December 29, 2006), http://www.cdc.gov/nchs/data/ad/ad381.pdf.
4. "Eczema Prevalence in the United States," National Eczema Association, accessed March 3, 2016, https://nationaleczema.org/research/eczema-prevalence.
5. CCFA, "Crohn's Disease & Ulcerative Colitis: A Guide for Parents," Crohn's & Colitis Foundation, accessed March 3, 2016, http://www.ccfa.org/resources/guide-for-parents.html.
6. "Celiac Disease: Fast Facts," Beyond Celiac, accessed July 6, 2016, http://www.beyondceliac.org/celiac-disease/facts-and-figures. Between 133 and 144 in different populations. Alberto Rubio-Tapia et al., "The Prevalence of Celiac Disease in the United States," American Journal of Gastroenterology 107, no. 10 (October 2012): 1538–44, doi:10.1038/ajg.2012.219. Finally, see: Michael A. D'Amico et al., "Presentation of Pediatric Celiac Disease in the United States: Prominent Effect of Breastfeeding," Clinical Pediatrics 44, no. 3 (April 2005), doi:10.1177/000992280504400309.

7. "Kids' Reflux—the Facts and the Stats," Reflux Infants Support Association, accessed July 7, 2016, http://www.reflux.org.au/information/kids-reflux-the-facts-and-the-stats; "Pediatric GERD (Gastro-Esophageal Reflux Disease)," American Academy of Otolaryngology—Head and Neck Surgery, accessed March 3, 2016, http://www.entnet.org/content/pediatric-gerd-gastro-esophageal-reflux-disease.
8. "Irritable Bowel Syndrome (IBS) in Children," National Institute of Diabetes and Digestive and Kidney Diseases, posted June 2014, accessed July 7, 2017, https://www.niddk.nih.gov/health-information/health-topics/digestive-diseases/ibs-in-children/Pages/facts.aspx.
9. Ebe D' Adamo and Sonia Caprio, "Type 2 Diabetes in Youth: Epidemiology and Pathophysiology," Diabetes Care 34, Suppl 2 (May 2011): S161–65, doi:10.2337/dc11-s212.
10. "Autism Prevalence," Autism Speaks, accessed March 3, 2016, https://www.autismspeaks.org/what-autism/prevalence.
11. "Attention-Deficit / Hyperactivity Disorder (ADHD): Data & Statistics," Centers for Disease Control and Prevention, accessed March 30, 2017, https://www.cdc.gov/ncbddd/adhd/data.html.
12. "Any Disorder among Children," National Institute of Mental Health, accessed March 3, 2017, http://www.nimh.nih.gov/health/statistics/prevalence/any-disorder-among-children.shtml.
13. Ishaq Abu-Arafeh et al., "Prevalence of Headache and Migraine in Children and Adolescents: A Systematic Review of Population-Based Studies," Developmental Medicine and Child Neurology 52, no. 12 (December 2010): 1088–97, doi:10.1111/j.1469-8749.2010.03793.
14. Vincanne Adams, Markets of Sorrow, Labors of Faith: New Orleans in the Wake of Katrina (Durham, NC: Duke University Press, 2013).

Chapter One: The Perfect Storm of Toxic Food, Sick Kids, and the Limits of Medicine

1. Jenny Perkel, "Parenting a Sick Child," Children in Mind (blog), posted June 6, 2011, accessed June 6, 2017, http://jennyperkel.com/parenting-a-sick-child.
2. All names of patients and their families, as well as physicians, are pseudonyms, and some genders have been changed to protect the privacy of persons whose stories appear here. IRB consent procedures for gathering the stories of these patients were obtained through Sutter Health and UCSF.
3. E. J. Mundell and HealthDay Reporter, "Rise in Child Chronic Illness Could Swamp Health Care," HealthDay ABC News, posted May 23, 2016, accessed July 9, 2016, http://abcnews.go.com/Health/Healthday/story?id=4507708&page=1.

Chapter Two: Going Beyond the Band-Aid to Help Chronically Sick Kids

1. For those interested in homeopathy, it is a medical science developed by Dr. Samuel Hahnemann in the late eighteenth century, early nineteenth century, based on the principle that "like cures like." In simple terms, it means that a substance that can produce symptoms that mimic the disease in a healthy person will, in extremely small doses, cure a patient who has those symptoms. There is much controversy about the effectiveness of homeopathy. For instance, the NIH is fairly negative: https://nccih.nih.gov/health/homeopathy. Many critics argue that effectiveness is largely based on placebo effect and that the dilution in these remedies is so small as to be clinically insignificant or, in short, nothing more than sugar pills. However, there are many supporters and a group of clinicians who are avid supporters of the practice and are unflinchingly convinced of its utility and effectiveness: https://homeopathic.com/category/homeopathic-research. For more information from a source that is positive about homeopathy, see Dana Ullman: http://www.homeopathic.com.

Chapter Three: Food-Focused Medicine for a Pharmaceutical-Heavy World

1. Kevin Quealy and Margot Sanger-Katz, "Is Sushi 'Healthy'? What about Granola? Where Americans and Nutritionists Disagree," New York Times, July 5, 2016, http://www.nytimes.com/interactive/2016/07/05/upshot/is-sushi-healthy-what-about-granola-where-americans-and-nutritionists-disagree.html.
2. Sarah Klein, "A Brief History of How Breakfast Got Its 'Healthy' Rep," Huffington Post, October 6, 2014, http://www.huffingtonpost.com/2014/10/06/breakfast-most-important-history_n_5910054.html.
3. James Harvey Young, The Medical Messiahs: A Social History of Health Quackery in 20th Century America (New Jersey: Princeton University Press, 2015).
4. Paul Starr, The Social Transformation of American Medicine: The Rise of a Sovereign Profession and the Making of a Vast Industry (New York: Basic Books, 1984).
5. For more on the peculiar and specific cultural construction of American modern medicine, or biomedicine from anthropological perspectives, see Deborah Gordon and Margaret M. Lock, Biomedicine Examined (Boston: Kluwer Academic Publisher, 1988), along with numerous other works.
6. Joseph Dumit, Drugs for Life (Durham: Duke University Press, 2012).
7. Hilary A. Tindle et al., "Trends in Use of Complementary and Alternative Medicine by US Adults: 1997–2002," Alternative Therapies in Health and Medicine11, no. 1(January/February 2005): 42–49, https://www.ncbi.nlm.nih.gov/pubmed/15712765.

8. For example, see "Alternative Medicine," Wikipedia, https://en.wikipedia.org/wiki/Alternative_medicine, accessed July 6, 2016. Integrative health centers are making a huge impact on how medicine perceives of the task of thinking beyond conventional biomedicine. The improved reception of integrative medicine and the degree to which medical centers will pay for it is being driven in part by the rise in people with complex chronic disorders. Thanks to Lindsay Berkowitz for her insights on this, as discussed in her UC Berkeley Sociology Master's thesis.
9. "Announcing the National Microbiome Initiative," The White House: President Barack Obama, accessed April 19, 2017, https://www.whitehouse.gov/blog/2016/05/13/announcing-national-microbiome-initiative.

Chapter Four: A Second Silent Spring

1. Jane Goodall, Harvest for Hope: A Guide to Mindful Eating (New York: Grand Central Publishing, 2006).
2. Michael Pollan, In Defense of Food: An Eater's Manifesto (New York: Penguin Press, 2008).
3. Sandra Steingraber, Raising Elijah: Protecting Our Children in an Age of Environmental Crisis (Philadelphia: De Capo, 2011).
4. David A. Kessler, The End of Overeating: Taking Control of the Insatiable American Appetite (New York: Rodale, 2010); Gary Taubes, The Case Against Sugar (New York: Alfred A. Knopf, 2016).
5. "The Story of Silent Spring," Natural Resource Defense Council, posted August 13, 2015, accessed March 21, 2016, https://www.nrdc.org/stories/story-silent-spring.
6. "FAQs on GE Crops," The National Academies of Sciences, Engineering, and Medicine, accessed March 21, 2016, http://nas-sites.org/ge-crops/2014/06/04/faq-on-ge-crops.
7. On the history of DDT politics: Elena Conis, "Debating the Health Effects of DDT: Thomas Jukes, Charles Wurster, and the Fate of an Environmental Pollutant," Public Health Reports 125, no. 2 (March/April 2010): 337–42, https://www.ncbi.nlm.nih.gov/pmc/articles/PMC2821864; Elena Conis, "DDT Disbelievers: Health and the New Economic Poisons in Georgia after World War II," Southern Spaces, October 28, 2016. On the shift from war industries to agroindustries: Steven Sadowsky, "Central Problem Rough Draft," Monsanto Papers, accessed online June 9, 2017, Monsanto Paper.docx – AGEC4433Team10.
8. Herbert Oberlander, "Howard A. Schneiderman: Planetary Patriot," American Zoologist 33, no. 3 (1993): 308–15. Another innovation that just preceded genetic modification was the development of an herbicide that was believed to be harmless to humans, called glyphosate, the active ingredient in Roundup (produced by Monsanto). We will hear more about this later.

9. B. A. Eskenazi, A. Bradman, and R. Castorina, "Exposures of Children to Organophosphate Pesticides and Their Potential Adverse Health Effects," Environmental Health Perspectives 107, Suppl 3 (June 1, 1999): 409–19, doi:10.1289/ehp.99107s3409.
10. Specifically, Eskenazi shows that organophosphate pesticides interfere with the enzyme that hydrolyzes/breaks down acetylcholine; thus it accumulates in high concentration at the neuronal junctions, which has different effects depending on the neuron fiber type (motor, central nervous, sympathetic, or parasympathetic). Acute symptoms of poisoning from these pesticides include a wide range of deleterious effects (including nausea and vomiting, lethargy, muscle weakness, tachycardia, hyporeflexia, hypertonia, and respiratory distress). It is important to note here that although glyphosate (which we will talk about in the next chapter) is classified as an organophosphate because it contains carbon and phosphate, it apparently does not affect the nervous system the way organophosphate insecticides do by inhibiting cholinesterase. However, this does not necessarily mean glyphosate is safe.
11. See the website for the Charge Study at http://beincharge.ucdavis.edu.
12. Alison Gemmill et al., "Residential Proximity to Methyl Bromide Use and Birth Outcomes in an Agricultural Population in California," Environmental Health Perspectives 121, no. 6 (June 2013): 737–43, doi:10.1289/ehp.1205682.
13. E. A. Guillette et al., "An Anthropological Approach to the Evaluation of Preschool Children Exposed to Pesticides in Mexico," Environmental Health Perspectives 106, no. 6 (June 1998): 347–53, http://www.ncbi.nlm.nih.gov/pmc/articles/PMC1533004.
14. "Atrazine," Pesticide Action Network, accessed July 7, 2016, http://www.panna.org/resources/atrazine.
15. Janette D. Sherman, "Chlorpyrifos (Dursban)-Associated Birth Defects: Report of Four Cases," Archives of Environmental Health 51, no. 1 (January/February 1996): 5–8, doi:10.1080/00039896.1996.9935986; Eric Lipton, "E.P.A. Chief, Rejecting Agency's Science, Chooses Not to Ban Insecticide," New York Times, March 29, 2017, https://www.nytimes.com/2017/03/29/us/politics/epa-insecticide-chlorpyrifos.html.
16. Eskenazi et al., "Exposures of Children to Organophosphate Pesticides."
17. Joseph Mercola, "Transgenic Wars—How GMOs Impact Livestock and Human Health around the Globe," Mercola, posted September 24, 2016, http://articles.mercola.com/sites/articles/archive/2016/09/24/transgenic-wars-gmo.aspx.
18. Åke Bergman et al., "The Impact of Endocrine Disruption: A Consensus Statement on the State of the Science," Environmental Health Perspectives 121, no. 4 (April 2013): A104–6, doi:10.1289/ehp.1205448.
19. Tracey J. Woodruff, Ami R. Zota, and Jackie M. Schwartz, "Environmental Chemicals in Pregnant Women in the United States: NHANES 2003–2004," Environmental Health Perspectives 119, no. 6 (June 2011): 878–85, doi:10.1289/ehp.100272. She also found high levels of polybrominated diphenyl ethers (PBDEs)

in twenty-five second-trimester pregnant women in California—the highest levels ever reported among pregnant women worldwide of banned chemicals used in flame retardants. This is likely the result of California's strict flammability regulations. PBDEs are persistent organic chemicals widely used as flame retardants in consumer products since the 1970s. The commercial mixtures are usually used in furniture, electronics, and other plastic products. Although PBDEs are being phased out, human exposure in the United States continues due to the slow replacement time of PBDE-containing products and ingestion of contaminated foods. "Study Finds High Levels of Flame Retardant Chemicals in California Pregnant Women," University of California San Francisco, News Center, August 10, 2011, accessed June 20, 2016, https://www.ucsf.edu/news/2011/08/10425/study-finds-high-levels-flame-retardant-chemicals-california-pregnant-women.

20. Patrice Sutton et al., "Reproductive Health and the Industrialized Food System: A Point of Intervention for Health Policy," Health Affairs 30, no. 5 (May 2011): 888–97, doi:10.1377/hlthaff.2010.1255. The online version of this article, along with updated information and services, is available at: http://content.healthaffairs.org/content/30/5/888.
21. Nicholas Kristof, "Contaminating Our Bodies with Everyday Products," New York Times, November 28, 2015, accessed June 5, 2017, http://www.nytimes.com/2015/11/29/opinion/sunday/contaminating-our-bodies-with-everyday-products.html. We also note that this passage has earlier origins. In 2008, Sharyle Patton of Commonweal stated it in a Newsweek article by Annie Underwood, "The Chemicals Within," Newsweek, January 26, 2008, http://www.newsweek.com/chemicals-within-87375; as did Bruce Lourie and Rick Smith in their book Toxin Toxout: Getting Harmful Chemicals Out of Our Bodies and Our World (New York: St. Martin's Press, 2014): 3.
22. Theo Colburn, Dianne Dumanoski, and John P. Myers, Our Stolen Future: Are We Threatening Our Fertility, Intelligence, and Survival?—A Scientific Detective Story (New York: Penguin Group, 1996): 35; Sara Mostafalou and Mohammad Abdollahi, "Pesticides: An Update of Human Exposure and Toxicity," Archives of Toxicology 91, no. 2 (February 2017), doi:10.1007/s00204-016-1849-x; Aimee Quitmeyer and Rebecca Roberts, "Babies, Bottles, and Bisphenol A: The Story of a Scientist-Mother," PLoS Biology 5, no. 7, e200 (July 2007): 1399–402, doi:10.1371/journal.pbio.0050200.
23. Steven M. Druker, Altered Genes, Twisted Truth: How the Venture Genetically Engineer our Food Has Substantially Subverted Science, Corrupted Government, and Systematically Deceived the Public (Salt Lake City, UT: Clear River Press, 2015).
24. Take the case of chlorpyrifos, an organophosphate pesticide. Chlorpyrifos was assigned a certain maximum level of exposure in June 2011. The levels reported in the general US population were seen to be roughly 0.009 micrograms of chlorpyrifos

per kilogram of body weight per day directly from food residue. Children were reported to have higher levels, at 0.025 micrograms. The EPA's acceptable daily dose was surprisingly higher than this, at 0.3 micrograms/kg/day. It was then reevaluated in December 2014 when it was realized to be more toxic than anticipated, and people were reporting health problems that were likely tied to exposure. The EPA finally responded by working with manufacturers to voluntarily restrict the use of chlorpyrifos in places where children might be exposed, including homes, schools, and day care centers. But it is still only marginally regulated as a pesticide. Even though there are voluntary limits set on its use for some crops, there is little done to control for problems of spray drift, so it is likely getting into much of the food supply. As with most pesticides, there are no studies of the long-term, cumulative, and augmentative effects of these chemicals in the context of multiple, concomitant chemical exposures. Again, the other problem with the EPA is that regulation efforts are only made in response to complaints, rather than concurrently with research efforts to find problems before they happen. J. D. Sherman, "Revised Human Health Risk Assessment on Chlorpyrifos," Environmental Protection Agency, accessed June 17, 2016, https://www.epa.gov/ingredients-used-pesticide-products/revised-human-health-risk-assessment-chlorpyrifos.

25. Joseph Mercola, "GMOs Should Be Banned: Found in 80% of Supermarket Foods," Mercola, posted May 20, 2011, accessed July 6, 2016, http://articles.mercola.com/sites/articles/archive/2011/05/20/most-evil-company-on-planet-soon-allowed-to-police-itself.aspx.
26. Another aspect of this turn to chemically rich agricultural strategies that could be explored is how they were part of the Green Revolution, the effort during the 1960s to do worldwide marketing of high-yield, high-fertilizer crops intended to solve world hunger problems.
27. Philip J. Landrigan and Charles Benbrook, "GMOs, Herbicides, and Public Health," New England Journal of Medicine 373 (2015): 693–95, doi:10.1056/NEJMp1505660.

Chapter Five: The Family Eating Modern Industrial Foods

1. Sharyle Patton of Commonweal quoted by Annie Underwood, "The Chemicals Within," Newsweek, January 26, 2008, http://www.newsweek.com/chemicals-within-87375.
2. Nicholas Kristof, "Contaminating Our Bodies with Everyday Products." Peter Turnbaugh's lab has shown that diet is by far the largest determinant and consistently resets and shapes the microbiome's composition in the short term and long term, but we still don't know much about how different kinds of food production might result in different microbial sustenance or harm. Conventional medical approaches argue that gluten-free diets don't have much impact on those who are

only suffering from Sjogren's who are not also celiac. But this viewpoint is being challenged.

3. A. Mosca et al., "Serum Uric Acid Concentrations and Fructose Consumption Are Independently Associated with NASH in Children and Adolescents," Journal of Hepatology 66, no. 5 (May 2017): 1031–36, doi:10.1016/j.jhep.2016.12.025.

Chapter Six: The Gut Microbiome, Symbiosis, and Dysbiosis

1. "Introduction to the Human Microbiome," American Microbiome Institute, accessed April 13, 2017, http://www.microbiomeinstitute.org/humanmicrobiome.
2. William Walsh, "Commentary on Nutritional Treatment of Mental Disorders," Safe Harbor, accessed July 6, 2017, http://www.alternativementalhealth.com /commentary-on-nutritional-treatment-of-mental-disorders-2.
3. Joshua Lederberg and Alexa T. McCray, "'Ome Sweet 'Omics—A Genealogical Treasury of Words," The Scientist 15, no. 7 (April 2, 2001): 8, https://lhncbc.nlm .nih.gov/files/archive/pub2001047.pdf; Jane Peterson et al., "The NIH Human Microbiome Project," Genome Research 19, no. 12 (December 2009): 2317–23, doi:10.1101/gr.096651.109.
4. Ron Sender, Shai Fuchs, Ron Milo, "Revised Estimates for the Number of Human and Bacteria Cells in the Body," PLoS Biology 14, no. 8 (August 19, 2016): e1002533, doi:10.1371/journal.pbio.1002533.
5. T. Yatsunenko et al., "Human Gut Microbiome Viewed across Age and Geography," Nature 468, no. 7402 (June 14, 2012): 222–27, doi:10.1038/nature 11053; see Jin Song et al., "Cohabiting Family Members Share Microbiota with One Another and with Their Dogs," eLife (2013): doi: 10.7554/eLife.00458.
6. From the research of B. Brett Finlay: Fredrik Backhed et al., "Defining a Healthy Human Gut Microbiome: Current Concepts, Future Directions, and Clinical Applications," Cell Host and Microbe 12, no. 5 (November 15, 2012): 611–22, doi:10.1016/j.chom.2012.10.012.
7. Toni Harman and Alex Wakeford, Your Baby's Microbiome: The Critical Role of Vaginal Birth and Breastfeeding for Lifelong Health (White River Junction, VT: Chelsea Green Publishing, 2017).
8. Maureen W. Groer et al., "Development of the Preterm Infant Gut Microbiome: A Research Priority," Microbiome 2 (2014): 38, doi:10.1186/2049-2618-2-38; Emily C. Gritz and Vineet Bhandari, "The Human Neonatal Gut Microbiome: A Brief Review," Frontier in Pediatrics 3 (March 5, 2015): 17, doi:10.3389/fped.2015.00017.
9. Mary Roach, Gulp: Adventures on the Alimentary Canal (New York: W. W. Norton, 2014).
10. Michael Pollan, "Some of My Best Friends Are Germs," New York Times Magazine, May 15, 2013, accessed July 11, 2016, http://www.nytimes.com/2013/05/19/magazine /say-hello-to-the-100-trillion-bacteria-that-make-up-your-microbiome.html.

11. Lynn Margulis, The Symbiotic Planet: A New Look at Evolution (New York: Basic Books, 2008). Others have commented on how this work offers a feminist reading of evolutionary science (for example, see Donna Haraway, Staying with the Trouble: Making Kin in the Chthulucene [Durham, NC: Duke University Press, 2016]).
12. Alex Vasquez, Human Microbiome and Dysbiosis in Clinical Disease: An Integrative Functional Medicine Approach to Understanding and Treating Microbial Imbalances and Chronic Infections, Volume 1: Parts 1–4 (International College of Human Nutrition and Functional Medicine, 2015).
13. Peris Mumbi Munyaka, Ehsan Khafipour, and Jean-Eric Ghia, "External Influence of Early Childhood Establishment of Gut Microbiota and Subsequent Health Implications," Frontier in Pediatrics 2 (2014): 109, doi:10.3389/fped.2014.00109.
14. Molly J. Stout et al., "Identification of Intracellular Bacteria in the Basal Plate of the Human Placenta in Term and Preterm Gestations," American Journal of Obstetrics and Gynecology 208, no. 3 (March 2013): 226, doi:10.1016/j.ajog.2013.01.018. Other articles of interest: Munyaka et al., "External Influence of Early Childhood Establishment of Gut Microbiota"; Kjersti Aagaard et al., "The Placenta Harbors a Unique Microbiome," Science Translation Medicine 6, no. 273 (May 21, 2014): 237–65, doi:10.1126/scitranslmed.3008599; Yann Fardini et al., "Transmission of Diverse Oral Bacteria to Murine Placenta: Evidence for the Oral Microbiome as a Potential Source of Intrauterine Infection," Infection and Immunity 78, no. 4 (April 2010): 1789–96, doi:10.1128/IAI.01395-09.
15. James J. Goedert et al., "Diversity and Composition of the Adult Fecal Microbiome Associated with History of Cesarean Birth or Appendectomy: Analysis of the American Gut Project," EBio Medicine 1, no. 2–3 (December 2014): 167–72, doi:10.1016/j.ebiom.2014.11.004.
16. Seppo Salminan and Erika Isolauri, "Opportunities for Improving the Health and Nutrition of the Human Infant by Probiotics," Nestle Nutrition Workshop Series, Pediatric Program 62 (2008): 223–33, doi:10.1159/000146350.
17. Jack A. Gilbert et al., "Toward Effective Probiotics for Autism and Other Neurodevelopmental Disorders," Cell 155, no. 7 (December 2013): 1446–48, doi:10.1016/j.cell.2013.11.035.
18. Backhed et al., "Defining a Healthy Human Gut Microbiome."
19. Evelien Neis, Cornelis H. C. Dejong, and Sander Rensen, "The Role of Microbial Amino Acid Metabolism in Host Metabolism," Nutrients 7, no. 4 (April 16, 2015): 2930–46, doi:10.3390/nu7042930; Meredith A. J. Hullar and Benjamin C. Fu, "Diet, the Gut Microbiome, and Epigenetics," Cancer Journal 20, no. 3 (May/June 2014): 170–75, doi:10.1097/PPO.0000000000000053; María Carmen Cenit et al., "Gut Microbiota and Attention Deficit Hyperactivity Disorder: New Perspectives for a Challenging Condition," European Child and Adolescent Psychiatry (March 13, 2017): 1–12, doi:10.1007/s00787-017-0969-z.

20. Augusto J. Montiel-Castro et al., "The Microbiota–Gut–Brain Axis: Neurobehavioral Correlates, Health and Sociality," Frontiers in Integrative Neuroscience 7 (October 7, 2013): 70, doi:10.3389/fnint.2013.00070; Sue Grenham et al., "Brain–Gut–Microbe Communication in Health and Disease," Frontiers in Physiology 2 (December 7, 2011): 94, doi:10.3389/fphys.2011.00094.
21. Peter J. Turnbaugh et al., "An Obesity-Associated Gut Microbiome with Increased Capacity for Energy Harvest," Nature 444 (December 21, 2006): 1027–31, doi:10.1038/nature05414.
22. J. L. Sabenet al., "Maternal Metabolic Syndrome Programs Mitochondrial Dysfunction via Germline Changes across Three Generations," Cell Reports 16/1 (2016): 1–8, doi:10.1016/j.celrep.2016.05.065.
23. J. L. Round and S. K. Mazmanian, "The Gut Microbiota Shapes Intestinal Immune Responses during Health and Disease," *Nature Reviews Immunology* 9 (May 2009): 313–323, doi:10.1038/nri2515; Vasquez, Human Microbiome and Dysbiosis in Clinical Disease.
24. Xing Hua et al., "Allergy Associations with the Adult Fecal Microbiota: Analysis of the American Gut Project," EBioMedicine 3 (November 27, 2016): 172–79, doi:10.1016/j.ebiom.2015.11.038.
25. Jun Chen et al., "Multiple Sclerosis Patients Have a Distinct Gut Microbiota Compared to Healthy Controls," Scientific Reports 6 (2016): 28484, doi:10.1038/srep28484.
26. Backhed et al., "Defining a Healthy Human Gut Microbiome."
27. Katherine Harmon Courage, "Fiber-Famished Gut Microbes Linked to Poor Health," Scientific American, March 23, 2015, accessed July 30, 2016, http://www.scientificamerican.com/article/fiber-famished-gut-microbes-linked-to-poor-health1.
28. Ian H. McHardy et al., "Integrative Analysis of the Microbiome and Metabolome of the Human Intestinal Mucosal Surface Reveals Exquisite Inter-relationships," Microbiome 1, no. 1 (2013): 17, doi:10.1186/2049-2618-1-17.
29. Lawrence A. David et al., "Diet Rapidly and Reproducibly Alters the Human Gut Microbiome," Nature 505 (January 23, 2014): 559–63, doi:10.1038/nature12820.
30. R. N. Carmody et al, "Diet Dominates Host Genotype in Shaping the Murine Gut Microbiota," Cell Host and Microbe 17, no. 1 (January 14, 2015): 72–84, doi:10.1016/j.chom.2014.11.010; David et al., "Diet Rapidly and Reproducibly Alters the Human Gut Microbiome."
31. Turnbaugh et al., "An Obesity-Associated Gut Microbiome with Increased Capacity for Energy Harvest"; Leslie Pray et al., The Human Microbiome, Diet, and Health: Workshop Summary (Washington, DC: The National Academies, 2013): 69–78.
32. Amy Langdon, Nathan Crook, and Gautam Dantas, "The Effects of Antibiotics on the Microbiome throughout Development and Alternative Approaches

for Therapeutic Modulation," Genome Medicine 8, no. 1 (April 13, 2016): 39, doi:10.1186/s13073-016-0294-z.

33. Pray et al., The Human Microbiome, Diet, and Health, 8. Cited in this passage is work from Gerard D. Wright, "The Antibiotic Resistome: The Nexus of Chemical and Genetic Diversity," Nature Reviews Microbiology 5, no. 3 (2007): 175–86, doi:10.1038/nrmicro1614.
34. Benoit Chassaing et al., "Dietary Emulsifiers Impact the Mouse Gut Microbiota Promoting Colitis and Metabolic Syndrome," Nature 519, no. 7541 (March 5, 2015): 92–96, doi:10.1038/nature14232.
35. Matam Vijay-Kumar et al., "Metabolic Syndrome and Altered Gut Microbiota in Mice Lacking Toll-Like Receptor 5," Science 328, no. 5975 (April 9, 2010): 228–31, doi:10.1126/science.1179721.
36. Pollan, "Some of My Best Friends Are Germs" (see n. 10).
37. Yatsunenko et al., "Human Gut Microbiome" (see n. 5).
38. Of course, there is also research pointing to the ways microbial communities can be harmed even by some organic foods, such as in a small number of plants whose natural toxins are produced to defend against pests in the absence of man-made pesticides. Researchers have argued for the benefits of pesticides in order to prevent our foods from becoming more toxin-rich. For instance, lectins in potatoes that are green, or the lining of cashew nut that must be cleaned off before it is edible. This is a problem that is uncommon, easily rectified by food preparation knowledge, and quite small in contrast to the amount of toxicants that are regularly put into most nonorganic foods. Maanvi Singh, "Can We Eat Our Way to a Healthier Microbiome? It's Complicated," NPR, The Salt: What's on Your Plate?, November 8, 2013, accessed June 5, 2017, http://www.npr.org/sections/thesalt/2013/11/08/243929866/can-we-eat-our-way-to-a-healthier-microbiome-its-complicated. See also: Rae Ellen Bichell, "When Edible Plants Turn Their Defense on Us," NPR, The Salt: What's on Your Plate?, October 23, 2013, accessed June 7, 2017, http://www.npr.org/blogs/thesalt/2013/10/01/228221063/when-edible-plants-turn-their-defenses-on-us.
39. Pray et al., The Human Microbiome, Diet, and Health.

Chapter Seven: Unconventional Medicine for Treating Gut Dysfunction

1. Of painful conditions in children, the number one cause is abdominal pain, and usually this is related to gastrointestinal problems. See Mark I. Neuman, "Causes of Acute Abdominal Pain in Children and Adolescents," UpToDate, last updated April 12, 2016, accessed October 10, 2016, http://www.uptodate.com/contents/causes-of-acute-abdominal-pain-in-children-and-adolescents.
2. This understanding of IgG and IgA immune reactions is debated. It is one of the areas of medicine that needs more research. For Dr. Perro, clinical and

laboratory evidence that such responses go away after the gut is healed, even after the offending foods are eaten again, suggests that even IgG and IgA need to be treated as pathological immune reactions rather than normal/healthy reactions. Other indications that these immune reactions should be used diagnostically are that family members eating the same foods show different levels of reactions, with the sickest members showing the highest levels of IgG and IgA antibodies to certain foods. For one side of the controversy, see Meghan Kemnec, "Understanding Food Allergy and Food Sensitivity (IgA vs IgG vs IgE reactions)," Naturopathic Pediatrics, posted February 10, 2017, http://naturopathicpediatrics.com/2017/02/10/understanding-food-allergy-food-sensitivity-iga-igg-ige. For the view that is critical of this argument, see Steven O. Stapel et al., "Testing for IgG4 against Foods Is Not Recommended as a Diagnostic Tool: EAACI Task Force Report," Allergy 63, no. 7 (July 2008): 793–96, doi:10.1111/j.1398-9995.2008.01705.x.

3. German Biological Medicines are a homeopathic formulary, not a brand. These remedies clean out and restore the extracellular matrix. For more on German Biological Medicines: Peter W. Gosch, Vital Energy Medicine: Using PEKANA Homeopathic-Spagyric Medications in the Tradition of German Complementary Medicine (Provo, UT: Chronicle Publishing Services, 2003).

Chapter Eight: Leaky Gut

1. John Swansburg, "Cute Family. And You Should See Their Bacteria," Science of Us, April 23, 2015, accessed June 17, 2016, http://nymag.com/scienceofus/2015/04/sonnenburg-family-stomach-bacteria.html.
2. Emily Martin, Flexible Bodies: Tracking Immunity in American Culture from the Days of Polio to the Age of AIDS (Boston: Beacon Press, 1994).
3. Martin also explored how these metaphors have changed over time. In fact, for most people living in industrialized countries during the last third of the twentieth century, such metaphors are no longer appropriate. Not only do they perpetuate stereotypes of our worst political principles (keeping out enemy forces and killing them to ensure this; characterizing them as "enemies" just because they are different), but such metaphors no longer work for the kinds of activities that are needed to keep us healthy. Indeed, because of antibiotics (as well as better sanitation, nutrition, and vaccines), diseases from infectious pathogens from TB to influenza are no longer causing the worst morbidities, at least not in wealthy and technologically advanced nations. We still need antibiotics and vaccines, but our more nefarious morbidities, including things that can kill us, according to Martin, are the chronic and persistent system malfunctions. These might have very little to do with infectious pathogens but a lot to do with our body's own reaction to survival in a world that is reaping the spoils of its own killing industries. Perhaps

chief among these are disorders in which the body's own immune system has turned against itself, the autoimmune disorders. Think of the rise in rates of inflammatory bowel disease, Type 2 diabetes, celiac disease, multiple sclerosis, rheumatoid arthritis, Hashimoto's thyroiditis—and then consider that the rates of these are going up for children.

4. Haraway, Staying with the Trouble (see chap. 6 n. 11).
5. Case Adams, Increased Intestinal Permeability, aka Leaky Gut Syndrome: The Science of Achieving Digestive Health (Wilmington, DE: Logical Books, 2012).
6. These are HLA-DQ2 and HLA-DQ8.
7. "Autoimmune diseases are characterized by tissue damage and loss of function due to an immune response that is directed against specific organs. This review is focused on the role of impaired intestinal barrier function on autoimmune pathogenesis. Together with the gut-associated lymphoid tissue and the neuroendocrine network, the intestinal epithelial barrier, with its intercellular tight junctions, controls the equilibrium between tolerance and immunity to non-self antigens. Zonulin is the only physiologic modulator of intercellular tight junctions described so far that is involved in trafficking of macromolecules and, therefore, in tolerance/immune response balance. When the zonulin pathway is deregulated in genetically susceptible individuals, autoimmune disorders can occur. This new paradigm subverts traditional theories underlying the development of these diseases and suggests that these processes can be arrested if the interplay between genes and environmental triggers is prevented by re-establishing the zonulin-dependent intestinal barrier function. Both animal models and recent clinical evidence support this new paradigm and provide the rationale for innovative approaches to prevent and treat autoimmune diseases." Alessio Fasano, "Leaky Gut and Autoimmune Diseases," Clinical Reviews in Allergy and Immunology 42, no. 1 (February 2012): 71–78, doi:10.1007/s12016-011-8291-x.
8. Ivor Hill et al., "The Prevalence of Celiac Disease in At-Risk Groups of Children in the United States," Journal of Pediatrics 136, no. 1 (January 2000): 86–90, doi:10.1016/S0022-3476(00)90055-6.
9. Melanie Uhde et al., "Intestinal Cell Damage and Systemic Immune Activation in Individuals Reporting Sensitivity to Wheat in the Absence of Coeliac Disease," Gut 65, no. 12 (July 25, 2016): 1921–22, doi:10.1136/gutjnl-2016-311964. For more on this topic: Columbia University Medical Center, "Biological Explanation for Wheat Sensitivity Found," Science Daily, posted July 26, 2016, https://www.sciencedaily.com/releases/2016/07/160726123632.htm.
10. Marilyn Hair and John Sharpe, "Fast Facts about the Human Microbiome," Center for Ecogenetics and Environment Health, January 2014, accessed July 30, 2016, http://depts.washington.edu/ceeh/downloads/FF_Microbiome.pdf.

11. On bacterial endotoxins: Kenneth Todar, "Bacterial Endotoxin," Todar's Online Textbook of Bacteriology, http://textbookofbacteriology.net/endotoxin.html.

Chapter Nine: Chronic Exposure

1. Steingraber, Raising Elijah, 46 (see chap. 4 no. 3).
2. Martin J. Blaser, MD, Missing Microbes: How the Overuse of Antibiotics Is Fueling Our Modern Plagues (New York: Henry Holt and Company, 2014); Moises Velasquez-Manoff, "The Parasite Underground," New York Times Magazine, June 16, 2016, http://www.nytimes.com/2016/06/19/magazine/the-parasite-underground.html. His book, An Epidemic of Absence: A New Way of Understanding Allergies and Autoimmune Diseases (New York: Scribner, 2012), is also useful on this topic.
3. Interestingly, the Amish do not do much organic farming, but it is not clear how much spraying they do nor is it clear that they predominantly use GM crops. Moises Velasquez-Manoff, "Health Secrets of Amish," New York Times, August 3, 2016, http://www.nytimes.com/2016/08/04/opinion/health-secrets-of-the-amish.html.
4. Steingraber, Raising Elijah, 46 (see chap. 4 no. 3).

Chapter Ten: The Making of Modern Industrialized Food

1. "Industrial Agriculture: The Outdated, Unsustainable System That Dominates U.S. Food Production," Union of Concerned Scientists, accessed April 19, 2017, http://www.ucsusa.org/our-work/food-agriculture/our-failing-food-system/industrial-agriculture.
2. Belinda Martineau, First Fruit (Chicago: Donnelly and Sons, 2001).
3. "Percentage of Genetically Modified Crops in the U.S. in 1997 and 2016, by Type (as Percent of Total Acreage)," Statista, accessed April 6, 2016, https://www.statista.com/statistics/217108/level-of-genetically-modified-crops-in-the-us; "Sugar & Sweeteners: Background," United States Department of Agriculture, accessed April 6, 2016, https://www.ers.usda.gov/topics/crops/sugar-sweeteners/background; Stanley R. Johnson et al., Quantification of the Impacts on US Agriculture of Biotechnology-Derived Crops Planted in 2006 (Washington, DC: National Center for Food and Agricultural Policy, 2008), accessed August 12, 2016, http://www.ncfap.org/documents/2007biotech_report/Quantification_of_the_Impacts_on_US_Agriculture_of_Biotechnology_Executive_Summary.pdf.
4. See the work of Center for Food Safety, and the documentary, Pesticides in Paradise, http://www.centerforfoodsafety.org/video.
5. Milk from these cows contains higher levels of IGF-1, which has been linked to cancer and Type I diabetes. The milk might also contain more pus (white blood

cells), since injecting cows with this hormone leads to higher levels of mastitis (and also lameness).

6. The Institute for Responsible Technology provides a list of foods that might contain GM ingredients. "GMOs in Food," Institute for Responsible Technology, accessed August 5, 2016, https:/responsibletechnology.org/gmo-education/gmos-in-food. For the reference to wine yeasts: Jamie Goode, "GM Yeasts: The Next Battleground," Wine Anorak, accessed June 8, 2017, http://www.wineanorak.com/GM_yeasts.htm.
7. Clive James, Global Status of Commercialized Biotech/GM Crops (Ithaca, NY: ISAAA, 2014), accessed June 7, 2017, http://www.isaaa.org/resources/publications/briefs/49/default.asp.
8. To date, there are no marketed versions of GM wheat; however, some "volunteer" GM strains of wheat have been found in at least three locations in the United States, one of which was a field that was formerly used for testing a version of GM wheat. "Detection of GE Wheat Volunteer Plants in Washington State," United States Department of Agriculture, last modified December 1, 2016, accessed June 7, 2017 https://www.aphis.usda.gov/aphis/ourfocus/biotechnology/brs-news-and-information/ge+wheat+washington+state.
9. The GMO Answers website (which is industry-sponsored) offers an explanation for why this company has a patent on this product as an antibiotic, but also claims it has no relationship to the problems of antibiotic resistance in clinical medicine: "Why Did Monsanto Patent Glyphosate as an Antibiotic?" question submitted by Transparency, response by Dan Goldstein, https://gmoanswers.com/ask/why-did-monsanto-patent-glyphosate-antibiotic-also-medical-establishment-has-been-preaching.
10. Charles M. Benbrook, "Impacts of Genetically Engineered Crops on Pesticide Use in the U.S.—the First Sixteen Years," Environmental Sciences Europe 24 (2012): 24, doi:10.1186/2190-4715-24–24; Doug Gurian-Sherman, Failure to Yield: Evaluating the Performance of Genetically Engineered Crops (Cambridge, MA: UCS Publications, 2009), accessed June 8, 2107, http://www.ucsusa.org/assets/documents/food_and_agriculture/failure-to-yield.pdf; and National Academies of Sciences, Engineering, and Medicine, Genetically Engineered Crops: Experiences and Prospects (Washington, DC: The National Academies Press, 2016).
11. Jeorg Graf, "Shifting Paradigm on Bacillus thuringiensis Toxin and a Natural Model for Enterococcus faecalis Septicemia," MBio 2, no. 4 (August 16, 2011): e00161-11, doi:10.1128/mBio.00161-1.
12. Matthias Meier and Angelika Hilbeck, "Influence of Transgenic Bacillus thuringiensis Corn-Fed Prey on Prey Preference of Immature Chrysoperla carnea (Neuroptera: Chrysopidae)," Basic and Applied Ecology 2, no. 1 (2001): 35–44, doi:10.1078/1439-1791-00034; J. E. Schmidt et al., "Effects of Activated

Bt Transgene Products (Cry1Ab, Cry3Bb) on Immature Stages of the Ladybird Adalia bipunctata in Laboratory Ecotoxicity Testing," Archives of Environmental Contamination and Toxicology 56, no. 2 (February 2009): 221–28, doi:10.1007/s00244-008-9191-9; Angelika Hilbeck et al., "A Controversy Re-visited: Is the Coccinellid Adalia bipunctata Adversely Affected by Bt Toxins?" Environmental Sciences Europe 24 (2012): 10, doi:10.1186/2190-4715-24-10; Angelika Hilbeck, Matthias Meier, and Miluse Tritkova, "Underlying Reasons of the Controversy over Adverse Effects of Bt Toxins on Lady Beetle and Lacewing Larvae," Environmental Sciences Europe 24 (2012): 9, doi:10.1186/2190-4715-24-9.

13. "Myth: GM Bt Crops Only Affect Target Pests and Their Relatives," Earth Open Source, accessed June 7, 2017, http://earthopensource.org/gmomythsandtruths/sample-page/5-gm-crops-impacts-farm-environment/5-4-myth-gm-bt-crops-affect-target-pests-relatives.
14. Margaret Douglas and John Tooker, "Large-Scale Deployment of Seed Treatments Has Driven Rapid Increase in Use of Neonicotinoid Insecticides and Preemptive Pest Management in U.S. Field Crops," Environmental Science and Technology 49, no. 8 (2015): 5088–97, doi:10.1021/es506141g.
15. András Székács and Béla Darvas, "Comparative Aspects of Cry Toxin Usage in Insect Control," chap. in Isaac Ishaaya, Subba Reddy Palli, A. Rami Horowitz, eds. Advanced Technologies for Managing Insect Pests (Netherlands: Springer, 2013), 195–230.
16. Aziz Aris and Samuel LeBlanc, "Maternal and Fetal Exposure to Pesticides Associated to Genetically Modify Foods in Eastern Townships of Quebec, Canada" Reproductive Toxicology 31, no. 4 (May 2011): 528–33, doi:10.1016/j.reprotox.2011.02.004.
17. C. Robinson et.al., "GMO Myths and Truths: 2nd Edition," Earth Open Source, accessed June 7, 2017, http://earthopensource.org/earth-open-source-reports/gmo-myths-and-truths-2nd-edition/.
18. Compositional studies and animal studies show (respectively) that Bt crops are not substantially or biologically equivalent to non-Bt counterparts. For compositional studies: L. Zolla et al., "Proteomics as a Complementary Tool for Identifying Unintended Side Effects Occurring in Transgenic Maize Seeds as a Result of Genetic Modifications," Journal of Proteome Research 7, no. 5 (May 2008): 1850–61, doi:10.1021/pr0705082; and E. M. Abdo, O. M. Barbary, and O. E. Shaltout, "Chemical Analysis of Bt Corn 'Mon-810: Ajeeb-YG®' and Its Counterpart Non-Bt Corn 'Ajeeb,'" IOSR Journal of Applied Chemistry 4, no. 1 (March–April 2013): 55–60, accessed June 7, 2017, http://iosrjournals.org/iosr-jac/papers/vol4-issue1/L0415560.pdf. For animal feeding studies: A. A. Gab-Alla et al., "Morphological and Biochemical Changes in Male Rats Fed on Genetically Modified Corn (Ajeeb YG)," Journal of American Science 8, no. 9 (2012): 1117–23,

accessed July 7, 2017, http://www.academia.edu/3138607/Morphological_and_Biochemical_Changes_in_Male_Rats_Fed_on_Genetically_Modified_Corn_Ajeeb_YG; Z. S. El-Shamei et al., "Histopathological Changes in Some Organs of Male Rats Fed on Genetically Modified Corn (Ajeeb YG)," Journal of American Science 8, no. 10 (2012): 684–96, accessed June 8, 2017, http://www.academia.edu/3405345/Histopathological_Changes_in_Some_Organs_of_Male_Rats_Fed_on_Genetically_Modified_Corn_Ajeeb_YG; Alberto Finamore et al., "Intestinal and Peripheral Immune Response to MON810 Maize Ingestion in Weaning and Old Mice," Journal of Agricultural and Food Chemistry 56, no. 23 (2008): 11533–39, doi:10.1021/jf802059w; Stine Kroghsbo et al., "Immunotoxicological Studies of Genetically Modified Rice Expressing PHA-E Lectin or Bt Toxin in Wistar Rats," Toxicology 245, no. 1–2 (March 12, 2008): 24–34, doi:10.1016/j.tox.2007.12.005.

19. Also, animal feeding studies and subsequent molecular analysis show harmful effects from Roundup Ready GM plants. For example: Manuela Malatesta et al., "A Long-Term Study on Female Mice Fed on a Genetically Modified Soybean: Effects on Liver Ageing," Histochemistry and Cell Biology 130, no. 5 (November 2008): 967–77, doi:10.1007/s00418-008-0476-x; Manuela Malatesta et al., "Fine Structural Analyses of Pancreatic Acinar Cell Nuclei from Mice Fed on Genetically Modified Soybean," European Journal of Histochemistry 47, no. 4 (October–December 2003): 385–88, accessed June 7, 2017, http://www.ejh.it/index.php/ejh/article/viewFile/851/971; M. Malatesta et al., "Ultrastructural Morphometrical and Immunocytochemical Analyses of Hepatocyte Nuclei from Mice Fed on Genetically Modified Soybean," Cell Structure and Function 27 (2002): 173–80, accessed June 7, 2017, http://stopogm.net/sites/stopogm.net/files/hepatocyte nucleimalatesta.pdf; L. Vecchio et al., "Ultrastructural Analysis of Testes from Mice Fed on Genetically Modified Soybean," European Journal of Histochemistry 48, no. 4 (October–December 2004): 448–54, https://www.ncbi.nlm.nih.gov/pubmed/15718213. The following study and subsequent molecular analysis show harmful effects from feeding Roundup Ready GM maize to rats: Gilles-Eric Séralini et al., "Republished Study: Long-Term Toxicity of a Roundup Herbicide and a Roundup-Tolerant Genetically Modified Maize," Environmental Sciences Europe 26 (2014): 14, doi:10.1186/s12302-014-0014-5; R. Mesnage et al., "Multiomics Reveal Non-Alcoholic Fatty Liver Disease in Rats Following Chronic Exposure to an Ultra-Low Dose of Roundup Herbicide," Scientific Reports 7 (2017): 39328, doi:10.1038/srep39328.
20. Joel Rosenblatt, Lydia Mulvany, and Peter Waldman, "EPA Official Accused of Helping Monsanto 'Kill' Cancer Study," Bloomberg, March 14, 2017, accessed April 6, 2017, https://www.bloomberg.com/news/articles/2017-03-14/monsanto-accused-of-ghost-writing-papers-on-roundup-cancer-risk.

21. The recent attack on Greenpeace, signed by Nobel laureates, is a good example of this. Joel Achenbach, "107 Nobel Laureates Sign Letter Blasting Greenpeace over GMOs," Washington Post, June 30, 2016, accessed October 11, 2016, https://www.washingtonpost.com/news/speaking-of-science/wp/2016/06/29/more-than-100-nobel-laureates-take-on-greenpeace-over-gmo-stance. On the other side, see the report by 230 concerned scientists on GMO safety: Rosenblatt et al., "EPA Official Accused of Helping Monsanto 'Kill' Cancer Study"; and see Angelika Hilbeck et al., "No Scientific Consensus on GMO Safety," Environmental Sciences Europe 27 (2015): 4, doi:10.1186/s12302-014-0034-1.
22. Backhed et al., "Defining a Healthy Human Gut Microbiome" (see chap. 6 n. 6).
23. Tom Laskawy, "Going Rogue: USDA May Have Just Opened the GMO Floodgates," Grist, July 12, 2011, http://grist.org/industrial-agriculture/2011-07-11-going-rogue-usda-may-have-just-opened-the-gmo-floodgates; "Restrictions on Genetically Modified Organisms: United States," Library of Congress, last modified June 9, 2015, https://www.loc.gov/law/help/restrictions-on-gmos/usa.php.
24. "U.S. Regulation of Genetically Modified Crops," Federation of American Scientists, accessed June 9, 2017, https://fas.org/biosecurity/education/dualuse-agriculture/2.-agricultural-biotechnology/us-regulation-of-genetically-engineered-crops.html; "Myth: GM Foods Are Strictly Tested and Regulated for Safety," Earth Open Source, accessed June 9, 2017, http://earthopensource.org/gmomythsandtruths/sample-page/2-science-regulation/2-1-myth-gm-foods-strictly-tested-regulated-safety; Druker, Altered Genes, Twisted Truth (chap. 4 n. 23).
25. Industry's own studies often show lack of equivalence but companies (and sometimes regulators) claim that the differences do not matter biologically. Here is an EFSA opinion showing this: Hans Christer Andersson, "Opinion of the Scientific Panel on Genetically Modified Organisms [GMO] Related to the Notification for the Placing on the Market of Insect Resistant Genetically Modified Maize Bt11, for Cultivation, Feed and Industrial Processing," European Food Safety Authority Journal 3, no. 5 (May 2005): 213, doi:10.2903/j.efsa.2005.213. For a detailed critique of how the FDA sidestepped and lied about the evidence on GM foods, see Druker, Altered Genes, Twisted Truth (chap. 4 n. 23).
26. For the regulatory overview, see "U.S. Regulation of Genetically Modified Crops" (see n. 24).
27. See "How Are GMO Foods Regulated?" GMO Answers, submitted by "aruss2010," response from Steve Savage, https://gmoanswers.com/ask/how-are-gmo-foods-regulated.
28. Gene editing offers a more robust and profound set of opportunities to do genetic modification. The health implications of these technologies are not yet known or studied. For more on gene editing, see Mali Prashant and Linzhao Cheng, "Concise

Review: Human Cell Engineering: Cellular Reprogramming and Genome Editing," Stem Cells 30, no. 1 (January 2012): 75–81, doi:10.1002/stem.735.

29. In the United States, activists have occasionally implemented bans on GMO crops, such as in several counties in California. The effort is small but growing.
30. The organophosphates include insecticides such as malathion, parathion, and chlorpyrifos.

Chapter Eleven: The GM-Food Debate

1. Cary Funk and Lee Rainie, "Public and Scientists' Views on Science and Society," Pew Research Center, January 29, 2015, accessed June 8, 2017, http://www.pewinternet.org/2015/01/29/public-and-scientists-views-on-science-and-society.
2. Gary Langer, "Poll: Skepticism of Genetically Modified Foods," ABC News, June 19, 2016, accessed July 9, 2016, http://abcnews.go.com/Technology/story?id=97567.
3. Glenn Davis Stone, "The Anthropology of Genetically Modified Crops," Annual Review of Anthropology *39* (October 2010): 381–400, http://www.annualreviews.org/doi/10.1146/annurev.anthro.012809.105058.
4. Sheldon Krimsky and Tim Schwab, "Conflicts of Interest among Committee Members in the National Academies' Genetically Engineered Crop Study," PLoS One 12, no. 2 (2017): e0172317, doi:10.1371/journal.pone.0172317.
5. Pamela J. Mink et al., "Epidemiologic Studies of Glyphosate and Non-cancer Health Outcomes: A Review," Regulatory Toxicology and Pharmacology 61, no. 2 (November 2011): 172–84, doi:10.1016/j.yrtph.2011.07.006.
6. "Distinction between Genetic Engineering and Conventional Plant Breeding Becoming Less Clear, Says New Report on GE Crops," National Academies of Sciences, Engineering, and Medicine, posted May 17, 2016, accessed June 9, 2017, http://www8.nationalacademies.org/onpinews/newsitem.aspx?RecordID=23395.
7. Gary Ruskin, "Jon Entine and Genetic Literacy Project Spin Chemical Industry PR," U.S. Right to Know, last modified July 18, 2017, accessed September 15, 2017, https://usrtk.org/hall-of-shame jon-entine-the-chemical-industrys-master-messenger/.
8. Beverly D. McIntyre et al,. eds., "Agriculture at a Crossroads: Synthesis Report," International Assessment of Agricultural Knowledge, Science and Technology for Development, 2009, accessed June 9, 2017, http://apps.unep.org/redirect.php?file=/publications/pmtdocuments/-Agriculture%20at%20a%20crossroads%20-%20Synthesis%20report-2009Agriculture_at_Crossroads_Synthesis_Report.pdf.
9. Philip Lymbery, "A Common Sense Approach to Feeding the World," Compassion in World Farming, accessed June 8, 2017, https://www.ciwf.org.uk/media/3758842/Food-Sense.pdf. Calculated from FAOSTAT online figures for global grain harvest (2009) and food value of cereals. Based on a calorific intake of 2,500 kcalories per person per day.

10. "SAVE FOOD: Global Initiative on Food Loss and Waste Reduction," Food and Agricultural Organization of the United Nations, accessed June 9, 2017, http://www.fao.org/save-food/en; "Organic vs Non-Organic Food," New Castle University, posted October 8, 2015, accessed June 9, 2017, http://www.ncl.ac.uk/press/news/2015/10/organicvsnon-organicfood; Marcin Barański et al., "Higher Antioxidant and Lower Cadmium Concentrations and Lower Incidence of Pesticide Residues in Organically Grown Crops: A Systematic Literature Review and Meta-Analyses," British Journal of Nutrition 112, no. 5 (September 14, 2014): 794–811, doi:10.1017/S0007114514001366.
11. Canadian Biotechnology Action Network, accessed June 5, 2017, http://www.cban.ca.
12. Rodale Institute, The Farming Systems Trial: Celebrating 30 Years, accessed September 16, 2017, www.rodaleinstitute.org/assets/FSTbookletFINAL.pdf.
13. Brown's Ranch, accessed June 9, 2017, http://brownsranch.us.
14. Greenpeace has been a vocal activist against golden rice: "'Golden' Rice: All Glitter, No Gold," Greenpeace, posted March 16, 2005, accessed October 12, 2016, http://www.greenpeace.org/international/en/news/features/failures-of-golden-rice; "The 'Golden Rice'—an Exercise in How Not to Do Science," Science in Society Archive, posted June 13, 2000, accessed October 12, 2016, http://www.i-sis.org.uk/rice.php. In early 2017, the International Rice Research Institute (IRRI), the entity rolling out Golden Rice, finally applied for permission to the Philippines' government to use the rice for food and feed. However, IRRI acknowledged that studies had not yet been performed to show that the rice was effective in reducing vitamin A deficiency. IRRI "What Is the Status of the Golden Rice Coordinated by IRRI?" accessed September 15, 2017," http://irri.org/golden-rice/faqs/what-is-the-status-of-the-golden-rice-project-coordinated-by-irri.
15. Canadian Biotechnology Action Network. See also Robinson, "GMO Myths and Truths" (see chap. 10 no. 17).
16. Canadian Biotechnology Action Network.
17. Kari Hammerschlag, Anna Lappé, and Stacy Malkan, Spinning Food: How Food Industry Front Groups and Covert Communications Are Shaping the Story of Food (Friends of the Earth, 2015), http://webiva-downton.s3.amazonaws.com/877/cb/5/6306/FOE_SpinningFoodReport_8-15.pdf.
18. Claire Robinson, Michael Antoniou, and John Fagan, GMO Myths and Truths: A Citizen's Guide to the Evidence on the Safety and Efficacy of Genetically Modified Crops (London: Earth Open Source, 2015).
19. For a film version of this, see Bertram Verhaag, Scientists under Attack: Genetic Engineering in the Magnetic Field of Money (Denkmal Film, 2010), DVD, 88 min.
20. Stanley W. B. Ewen and Arpad Pusztai, "Effect of Diets Containing Genetically Modified Potatoes Expressing Galanthus nivalis Lectin on Rat Small Intestine,"

The Lancet 354, no. 9187 (October 16, 1999): 1353–54, doi:10.1016/S0140-6736 (98)05860-7.

21. Also we credit Michael Antoniou and Claire Robinson for the wording in some of this section on Pusztai. See also Robinson et al., GMO Myths and Truths.
22. In the film The World According to Monsanto by Marie-Monique Robin, Pusztai states that the transgene was not the problem but rather the problem was the technology of genetic modification.
23. Andrew Rowell, Don't Worry, It's Safe to Eat: The True Story of GM Food, BSE, and Foot and Mouth (London: Earthscan Publications, 2003); Jeffrey Smith "Genetically Modified Foods and Dr. Arpad Pusztai," video, posted August 9, 2010, accessed June 9, 2017, https://www.bibliotecapleyades.net/ciencia/ciencia_geneticfood36.htm; "Why I Cannot Remain Silent: Interview with Dr Arpad Pusztai," GM-Free 1, no. 3 (August/September 1999), http://gmwatch.org/index.php?option=com_content&view=article&id=13856; "Arpad Pusztai," Powerbase, last modified June 6, 2014, accessed June 5, 2017, http://www.powerbase.info/index.php/Arpad_Pusztai; Andrew Rowell, "The Sinister Sacking of the World's Leading GM Expert and the Trail That Leads to Tony Blair and the White House," The Daily Mail, July 7, 2003, accessed June 8, 2017, http://www.gmwatch.org/latest-listing/42-2003/4305; and Verhaag, Scientists under Attack.
24. Thanks to Michael Antoniou and Claire Robinson, authors of GMO Myths and Truths, for specifics here.
25. Rowell, "The Sinister Sacking of the World's Leading GM Expert."
26. Morten Poulsen et al., "A 90-Day Safety Study in Wistar Rats Fed Genetically Modified Rice Expressing Snowdrop Lectin Galanthus nivalis (GNA)," Food and Chemical Toxicology 45, no. 3 (2007): 350–63, doi:10.1016/j.fct.2006.09.002.
27. Séralini et al., "Retracted: Long-term Toxicity of a Roundup Herbicide and a Roundup-tolerant Genetically Modified Maize," Food and Chemical Toxicology 50, no. 11 (November 2012): 4221–4231, https://doi.org/10.1016/j.fct.2012.08.005.
28. Gilles-Eric Séralini, Dominique Cellier, and Joël Spiroux de Vendomois, "New Analysis of a Rat Feeding Study with a Genetically Modified Maize Reveals Signs of the Hepatorenal Toxicity," Archives of Environmental Contamination and Toxicology 52, no. 4 (May 2007): 596–602, doi:10.1007/s00244-006-0149-5.
29. Séralini et al., "Republished Study: Long-Term Toxicity of a Roundup Herbicide" (see chap. 10 n. 19).
30. See also a review of the controversy: Ulrich E. Leoning, "A Challenge to Scientific Integrity: A Critique of the Critics of the GMO Rat Study Conducted by Gilles-Eric Séralini et al. (2012)," Environmental Sciences Europe 27 (2015): 13, doi:10.1186/s12302-015-0048-3.
31. "Monsanto Secret Documents Show Massive Secret Attack on Séralini Study," Sustainable Pulse, posted August 1, 2017, http://sustainablepulse.com/2017/08/01

/monsanto-secret-documents-show-massive-attack-on-seralini-study/#.
WYjOkMaZOi4.

32. GM Watch also offers a good review of the suspicious nature of the attacks. There is evidence varying from extensive to suggestive that the attacks on Pusztai and Séralini (along with two others we don't include here: Chapela and Quist) were orchestrated by industry. See, for example, the case of Quist/Chapela here: "Myth: Independent Studies Confirm That GM Foods and Crops Are Safe," Earth Open Source, accessed July 25, 2017, http://earthopensource.org/gmomythsandtruths/sample-page/2-science-regulation/2-2-myth-independent-studies-confirm-gm-foods-crops-safe. See also: Jonathan Matthews, "Smelling a Corporate Rat," Spin Watch, December 11, 2012, accessed June 9, 2017, http://www.spinwatch.org/index.php/issues/science/item/164-smelling-a-corporate-rat; Claire Robinson and Jonathan Latham, "The Goodman Affair: Monsanto Targets the Heart of Science," Independent Science News, posted May 20, 2013, accessed June 9, 2017, https://www.independentsciencenews.org/science-media/the-goodman-affair-monsanto-targets-the-heart-of-science. And on one Séralini attacker, Bruce Chassy, who failed to disclose Monsanto funding: "Prof Bruce Chassy Failed to Disclose Monsanto Funding," GM Watch, posted March 17, 2016, accessed June 9, 2017, http://www.gmwatch.org/news/latest-news/16806.
33. Aysun Kiliç and Mehmet Turan Akay, "A Three Generation Study with Genetically Modified Bt Corn in Rats: Biochemical and Histopathological Investigation," Food and Chemical Toxicology 46, no. 3 (March 2008): 1164–70, doi:10.1016/j.fct.2007.11.016.
34. See this study of Bt maize on immune systems of pigs by Judy Carman, whose work we will explore later: Maria C. Walsh et al., "Fate of Transgenic DNA from Orally Administered Bt MON810 Maize and Effects on Immune Response and Growth in Pigs," PLoS One 6, no. 11 (2011): e27177, doi:10.1371/journal.pone.0027177.
35. Ezequiel Adamovsky, "Andres Carrasco vs Monsanto," TeleSUR, posted October 1, 2014, accessed October 15, 2016, http://www.telesurtv.net/english/opinion/Andres-Carrasco-vs-Monsanto-20141001-0090.html.
36. Johanna Choumert and Pascale Phelinas, "Is GM Soybean Cultivation in Argentina Sustainable?" HAL Archives Ouvertes 14 (2016), https://halshs.archives-ouvertes.fr/halshs-01356209/document; Mike Ludwig, "War over Monsanto Gets Ugly," Truthout, November 9, 2010, http://www.truth-out.org/archive/component/k2/item/92751:war-over-monsanto-gets-ugly.
37. The authors have attended multiple workshops and retreats on GMO science where they were told these stories directly.
38. The list is long of outspoken individuals who have been made publicly controversial. Scientists include: Simon Hogan, Belinda Martineau, Stephanie Seneff, Nancy Swanson, and Thierry Vrain. Some of these scientists previously worked for industry

and then came out against it. Public activists and farmers include Zen Honeycutt, Jeffrey Smith, and Percy Schmeiser, among many others.

Chapter Twelve: Going with Our Glyphosate-Filled Gut

1. Joseph Mercola, "Sudden Death Syndrome: The Hidden Epidemic Destroying Your Gut Flora," Mercola, posted December 10, 2011, http://articles.mercola.com/sites/articles/archive/2011/12/10/dr-don-huber-interview-part-1.aspx.
2. Landrigan and Benbrook, "GMOs, Herbicides, and Public Health" (see chap. 4 n. 27). Another report says glyphosate use has increased 100-fold since the 1970s: John Peterson Myers et al., "Concerns over Use of Glyphosate-Based Herbicides and Risks Associated with Exposures: A Consensus Statement," Environmental Health 15 (2016): 19, doi:10.1186/s12940-016-0117-0.
3. "Glyphosate and Glyphosate-Based Herbicides," GMO Science, last modified January 21, 2016, https://www.gmoscience.org/glyphosate-based-herbicides.
4. Myers et al., "Concerns over Use of Glyphosate-Based Herbicides."
5. "Estimated Annual Agricultural Pesticide Use: Pesticide Use Maps—Glyphosate," US Geological Survey, last modified January 12, 2017, https://water.usgs.gov/nawqa/pnsp/usage/maps/show_map.php?year=2014&map=GLYPHOSATE&hilo=L&disp=Glyphosate.
6. GM Watch says: "The allowed level in teff animal feed will be 100 parts per million (ppm)." GM Watch, "Monsanto's Minions: US EPA Hikes Glyphosate Limits in Food and Feed Once Again," Organic Consumers Association, accessed August 5, 2016, https://www.organicconsumers.org/news/monsantos-minions-us-epa-hikes-glyphosate-limits-food-and-feed-once-again.
7. See this study, which has a "lay" explanation: Thomas Bøhn et al., "Compositional Differences in Soybeans on the Market: Glyphosate Accumulates in Roundup Ready GM Soybeans," Food Chemistry 153 (June 15, 2014): 207–15, doi:10.1016/j.foodchem.2013.12.054; Thomas Bøhn and Marek Cuhra, "How 'Extreme Levels' of Roundup in Food Became the Industry Norm," Independent Science News, posted March 24, 2014, accessed June 8, 2017, https://www.independentsciencenews.org/news/how-extreme-levels-of-roundup-in-food-became-the-industry-norm. Also see this report, which is self-explanatory: "High Levels of Residues from Spraying with Glyphosate Found in Soybeans in Argentina," Test Biotech 22 (2013): 10, http://www.testbiotech.org/sites/default/files/TBT_Background_Glyphosate_Argentina_0.pdf.
8. A report from the World Health Organization (updated in 2005, but based mostly on research done in the 1980s and 1990s) assuaged concerns about the presence of glyphosate in drinking water from its use on crops. Although they note that "one can find residues in air, drinking-water, crops and animal tissues destined for human consumption" it does not "bioaccumulate." They summarize that the

amounts of glyphosate (and its breakdown product AMPA) are transient and so this, coupled with the evidence that there was no toxicity from these levels of exposure, made it unnecessary for regulation at the time. World Health Organization, "Glyphosate and AMPA in Drinking-Water," accessed June 8, 2017, http://www.who.int/water_sanitation_health/dwq/chemicals/glyphosateampa290605.pdf. See also: Jeff Schuette, "Environmental Fate of Glyphosate," Environmental Monitoring & Pest Management, Department of Pesticide Regulation, last updated November 1998, http://www.cdpr.ca.gov/docs/emon/pubs/fatememo/glyphos.pdf.

9. For instance, these sites use this sort of language to claim the safety of this pesticide: "Experimental evidence has shown that neither glyphosate nor AMPA bioaccumulates in any animal tissue. No significant toxicity occurred in acute, subchronic, and chronic studies. . . . For purposes of risk assessment, no-observed-adverse-effect levels (NOAELs) were identified for all subchronic, chronic, developmental, and reproduction studies with glyphosate, AMPA, and POEA. As pesticides go, [they summarize] glyphosate has very low toxicity, and any dose a person is likely to get exposed to is well below the safety limits." Steven Novella, "Glyphosate—The New Bogeyman," Science-Based Medicine, posted December 31, 2014, https://www.sciencebasedmedicine.org/glyphosate-the-new-bogeyman.
10. Bøhn et al., "Compositional Differences in Soybeans on the Market"; Monika Kruger et al., "Field Investigations of Glyphosate in Urine of Danish Dairy Cows," Journal of Environmental and Analytical Toxicology 3, no. 5 (2013): 1–7, doi:10.4172/2161-0525.1000186.
11. The officially allowed maximum residue level (MRL) in wheat is 10 mg per kg, a limit that was set before the World Health Organization's International Agency for Research on Cancer found glyphosate is a probable carcinogen to humans. "Pesticides," Health and Safety Executive, accessed October 15, 2016, http://www.hse.gov.uk/pesticides/#bread_and_pasta.
12. Soil Association, Glyphosate in our Bread—Facts & Figures, July 2015, accessed September 13, 2017, https://archive.senseaboutscience.org/data/files/VoYS/Glyphosate_in_our_bread.pdf.
13. Alliance for Natural Health USA, "Glyphosate Found in Popular Breakfast Foods," Eco Watch, posted April 19, 2016, accessed October 15, 2016, http://www.ecowatch.com/glyphosate-found-in-popular-breakfast-foods-1891117855.html. This study used ELISA testing that has disputed accuracy. For a study that used the more reliable testing method (LC-MS/MS) and was performed by an accredited, FDA-registered lab and found also very high levels, see "Alarming Levels of Glyphosate Contamination Found in Popular American Foods," Sustainable Pulse, posted November 14, 2016, accessed September 15, 2017, http://sustainablepulse.com/2016/11/14alarming-levels-of-glyphosate-contamination-found-in-popular-american-foods/#.Wbkv14prxJw.

14. For urine: Axel Adams et al., "Biomonitoring of Glyphosate Across the United States in Urine and Tap Water Using High-Fidelity LC-MS/MS Method," (poster presented at the University of California San Francisco, accessible at "UCSF Presentation Reveals Glyphosate Contamination in People Across America," The Detox Project, posted May 25, 2016, accessed October 16, 2016, https://detoxproject.org/1321-2/); Lars Niemann et al., "A Critical Review of Glyphosate Findings in Human Urine Samples and Comparison with the Exposure of Operators and Consumers," Journal für Verbraucherschutz und Lebensmittelsicherheit 10, no. 1 (March 2015): 3–12, doi:10.1007/s00003-014-0927-3. For breast milk: Zen Honeycutt and Henry Rowlands, "Glyphosate Testing Full Report: Findings in American Mothers' Breast Milk, Urine and Water," Moms Across America, posted April 7, 2014, accessed August 5, 2016, http://www.momsacrossamerica.com/glyphosate_testing_results.
15. Adams et al., "Biomonitoring of Glyphosate across the United States."
16. Charles Benbrook et al., "Herbicide Use and Birth Outcomes in the Midwest," Children's Environmental Health Network, accessed April 10, 2016, http://cehn-healthykids.org/the-project/the-science-team/the-science-team-select-publications.
17. GM Freeze and Friends of the Earth, "Government Urged to Act after Weedkiller Traces Found in Britons," GM Freeze, posted June 13, 2013, accessed October 16, 2016, http://www.gmfreeze.org/news-releases/225.
18. Angelika Steinborn et al., "Determination of Glyphosate Levels in Breast Milk Samples from Germany by LC-MS/MS and GC-MS/MS," Journal of Agricultural and Food Chemistry 64, no. 6 (2016): 1414–1421. doi:10.1021/acs.jafc.5b05852; "Greens Warn: German Breast Milk Unsafe" posted June 27, 2015, accessed September 15, 2017, https://www.thelocal.de/20150626/concerns-over-safety-of-german-breast-milk.
19. Michelle K. McGuire et al., "Glyphosate and Aminomethylphosphonic Acid Are Not Detectable in Human Milk," American Journal of Clinical Nutrition 103, no. 5 (March 2016): 1285–90. doi:10.3945/ajcn.115.126854; Steinborn et al., "Determination of Glyphosate Levels in Breast Milk Samples."
20. Niemann et al., "A Critical Review of Glyphosate Findings in Human Urine Samples."
21. Set by the Joint FAO/WHO Meeting on Pesticide Residues, "Glyphosate," FAO, http://www.fao.org/docrep/w8141e/w8141e0u.htm.
22. Eskenazi et al., "Exposures of Children to Pesticides" (see chap. 4 n. 9).
23. D. W. Brewster, J. Warren, and W. E. Hopkins, 2nd, "Metabolism of Glyphosate in Sprague-Dawley Rats: Tissue Distribution, Identification, and Quantitation of Glyphosate-Derived Materials Following a Single Oral Dose," Fundamental and Applied Toxicology 17, no. 1 (July 1991): 43–51, https://www.ncbi.nlm.nih.gov

/pubmed/1916078. The EPA states allowable limits for animals and food crops in 2013: "The allowed level in teff animal feed will be 100 parts per million (ppm); and in oilseed crops, 40 ppm. Allowed levels in some fruits and vegetables eaten by humans will also rise: GM Watch, "Monsanto's Minions." Another source provides insight on the amount it changed in 2013: "Glyphosate levels in oilseed crops, which include sesame, flax, and soybean, from 20 parts per million (ppm), to 40 ppm. It also raises the allowable glyphosate contamination level for sweet potatoes and carrots from 0.2 ppm to 3 ppm for sweet potatoes and 5ppm for carrots, which are 15 and 25 times the previous levels." Laura Sesana, "EPA Raises Levels of Glyphosate Residue Allowed in Food," Washington Times, posted July 5, 2013, accessed June 7, 2017, http://gmoinside.org/epa-raises-levels-of-glyphosate-residue-allowed-in-food.

24. Siriporn Thongprakaisang et al., "Glyphosate Induces Human Breast Cancer Cell Growth via Estrogen Receptors," Food and Chemical Toxicology 59 (September 2013): 129–36, doi:10.1016/j.fct.2013.05.057.
25. N. Benachour et al., "Time- and Dose-Dependent Effects of Roundup on Human Embryonic and Placental Cells," Archives of Environmental Contamination and Toxicology 53, no. 1 (July 2007), 126–33, doi:10.1007/s00244-006-0154-8; Sophie Richard et al., "Differential Effects of Glyphosate and Roundup on Human Placental Cells and Aromatase," Environmental Health Perspectives 113, no. 6 (June 2005): 716–20, doi:10.1289/ehp.7728.
26. S. Guilhereme et al., "DNA Damage in Fish (Anguilla anguilla) Exposed to a Glyphosate-Based Herbicide—Elucidation of Organ-Specificity and the Role of Oxidative Stress," Mutation Research 743, no. 1–2 (March 2012): 1–9, doi:10.1016/j.mrgentox.2011.10.017.
27. Robin Mesnage et al., "Transcriptome Profile Analysis Reflects Rat Liver and Kidney Damage Following Chronic Ultra-Low Dose Roundup Exposure," Environmental Health 14 (2015): 70, doi:10.1186/s12940-015-0056-1. See also Myers et al., "Concerns over Use of Glyphosate-Based Herbicides" (see n. 4).
28. Mariana Astiz et al., "Overview of Glyphosate Toxicity and Its Commercial Formulations Evaluated in Laboratory Animal Tests," Current Topics in Toxicology 6 (2009): 1–15, accessed June 7, 2017, https://www.researchgate.net/publication/286532156_Overview_of_glyphosate_toxicity_and_its_commercial_formulations_evaluated_in_laboratory_animal_tests; Mariana Astiz, María J. T. de Alaniz, and Carlos Alberto Marra, "Effect of Pesticides on Cell Survival in Liver and Brain Rat Tissues," Ecotoxicology and Environmental Safety 72, no. 7 (October 2009): 2025–32, doi:10.1016/j.ecoenv.2009.05.001.
29. Mesnage et al., "Multiomics Reveal Non-Alcoholic Fatty Liver Disease" (see chap. 10 n. 19).
30. Allan E. Rettie and Jeffery P. Jones, "Clinical and Toxicological Relevance of CYP2C9: Drug-Drug Interactions and Pharmacogenetics," Annual Review of

Pharmacology and Toxicology 45 (January 2005): 477–94, doi:10.1146/annurev.pharmtox.45.120403.095821; C. J. Beuret, F. Cirulnik, and M. S. Gimnez, "Effect of the Herbicide Glyphosate on Liver Lipoperoxidation in Pregnant Rats and Their Fetuses," Reproductive Toxicology 19, no. 4 (March–April 2005): 501–4, doi:10.1016/j.reprotox.2004.09.009.

31. Robin Mesnage, B. Bernay, and G. E. Séralini, "Ethoxylated Adjuvants of Glyphosate-Based Herbicides Are Active Principles of Human Cell Toxicity," Toxicology 313, no. 2–3 (November 16, 2013): 122–28, doi:10.1016/j.tox.2012.09.006; Kathryn Z. Guyton et al., "Carcinogenicity of Tetrachlorvinphos, Parathion, Malathion, Diazinon, and Glyphosate," The Lancet: Oncology 16, no. 5 (May 2015): 490-91, doi:10.1016/S1470-2045(15)70134-8; Robin Mesnage et al., "An Integrated Multi-omics Analysis of the NK603 Roundup-Tolerant GM Maize Reveals Metabolism Disturbances Caused by the Transformation Process," Scientific Reports 6 (2016): 37855, doi:10.1038/srep37855.
32. Marie-Monique Robin, The World According to Monsanto: Pollution, Corruption, and the Control of the World's Food Supply (New York: The New Press, 2010): 81–3, who cites Julie Marc, "Effets toxiques d'herbicides à base de glyphosate sur la régulation du cycle cellulaire et le développement précoce en utlilisant l'embyron d'oursin," Toxicologie 1 (September 10, 2004).
33. Mesnage et al., "An Integrated Multi-omics Analysis of the NK603 Roundup-Tolerant GM Maize"; Séralini et al., "Republished Study: Long-Term Toxicity of a Roundup Herbicide" (see chap. 10 n. 19).
34. Awad Shehata et al., "The Effect of Glyphosate on Potential Pathogens and Beneficial Members of Poultry Microbiota in Vitro," Current Microbiology 66, no. 4 (2013): 350–358, doi:10.1007/s00284-012-0277-2.
35. Judy A. Carman et al., "A Long-Term Toxicology Study on Pigs Fed a Combined Genetically Modified (GM) Soy and GM Maize Diet," Journal of Organic Systems 8, no. 1 (2013): 38–54, accessed April 17, 2017, http://genera.biofortified.org/view/Carman2013. In personal correspondence with one author (Vlieger), we affirmed that they used both Roundup Ready and Bt maize as stacked traits in the test food sample.
36. Carman et al., "Long-Term Toxicology Study on Pigs." We also note that Dr. Carman believes she was attacked, with her website being targeted over thirty-five times, by enemies she assumes were industry-supported (personal communication). There is much spurious criticism of her work on the internet.
37. "Glyphosate Overview," GMO Free USA, accessed April 17, 2016, http://www.gmofreeusa.org/research/glyphosate/glyphosate-overview.
38. Shehata et al., "Effect of Glyphosate on Potential."
39. M. Rossi, A. Amaretti, and S. Raimondi, "Folate Production by Probiotic Bacteria," Nutrients 3, no. 1 (January 2011): 118–34. For references for the antibiotic effects

of glyphosate on animals, see the collection on Zotero, "Glyphosate Microbiota and Microbiomes," at https://www.zotero.org/groups/glyphosate_microbiota_and_microbiomes, accessed July 23, 2016. Claims of the health risks are contested by organizations like the Genetic Literacy Project: David Warmflash, "Glyphosate Used with GMO Crops under Attack for Disrupting Microbiome: Science or a Gut Feeling?" Genetic Literacy Project, posted December 5, 2014, accessed June 8, 2017, https://www.geneticliteracyproject.org/2014/12/05/glyphosate-used-with-gmo-crops-under-attack-for-disrupting-microbiome-science-or-a-gut-feeling.

40. A controversial effort to link glyphosate to these processes is: Anthony Samsel and Stephanie Seneff, "Glyphosate's Suppression of Cytochrome P450 Enzymes and Amino Acid Biosynthesis by the Gut Microbiome: Pathways to Modern Diseases," Entropy 15, no. 4 (2013): 1416–63, doi:10.3390/e15041416. Also, Myers et al., "Concerns over Use of Glyphosate-Based Herbicides" (see n. 2).
41. "Glyphosate and Glyphosate-Based Herbicides" (see n. 3). See also Kruger et al., "Field Investigations of Glyphosate in Urine of Danish Dairy Cows" (see n. 10).
42. Mesnage et al., "Ethoxylated Adjuvants of Glyphosate Based Herbicides"; see also: Mesnage et al., "Transcriptome Profile Analysis Reflects Rat Liver and Kidney Damage."
43. "High Glyphosate Levels in Mothers Leads to Shorter Pregnancies and Smaller Babies—New Ongoing Study," Sustainable Pulse, posted April 5, 2017, accessed June 8, 2017, http://sustainablepulse.com/2017/04/05/high-glyphosate-levels-in-mothers-leads-to-shorter-pregnancies-and-smaller-babies-new-ongoing-study.
44. "IARC Monographs Volume 112: Evaluation of Five Organophosphate Insecticides and Herbicides," World Health Organization, March 20, 2015, accessed June 9, 2017, https://www.iarc.fr/en/media-centre/iarcnews/pdf/MonographVolume112.pdf.
45. "Glyphosate to Be Listed under Proposition 65 as Known to the State to Cause Cancer," OEHHA, Science for a Healthy California, posted March 28, 2017, accessed June 9, 2017, https://oehha.ca.gov/proposition-65/crnr/glyphosate-be-listed-under-proposition-65-known-state-cause-cancer.
46. "IARC's Report on Glyphosate," Monsanto (website), posted April 21, 2017, accessed June 8, 2017, http://www.monsanto.com/iarc-roundup/pages/default.aspx.
47. "Ground Water and Drinking Water: National Primary Drinking Water Regulations," US EPA, accessed Sept. 15, 2017, https://www.epa.gov/ground-water-and-drinking-water/national-primary-drinking-water-regulations; "Glyphosate: General Fact Sheet," National Pesticide Information Center, accessed Sept 15, 2017, http://npic.orst.edu/factsheets/glyphogen.html; Laura Sesana, "Are EPA Approved Levels of Glyphosate Residues in Our Foods Too High?" Communities Digital News, posted April 6, 2014, accessed June 8, 2017, http://www.commdiginews.com/health-science/are-epa-approved-levels-of-glyphosate-residue-in-our-foods-too-high-13855.

48. "Secret Documents Show Monsanto Led Brutal Attack on International Cancer Agency," Sustainable Pulse, posted August 4, 2017, accessed September 16, 2017, http://sustainablepulse.com/2017/08/04/secret-documents-show-monsanto-behind-brutal-attack-on-international-cancer-agency/#.WYnWncaZPq0.
49. The Rodale Institute notes that non-GE soy had more protein and lower saturated fat levels compared to GE soy: for instance, Leah Zerbe, "Extreme Levels of Roundup Detected in Food," posted April 25, 2014, http://www.rodalesorganiclife.com/food/roundup-food. Antioxidants are also higher in non-GE foods (Claire Robinson, personal communication).
50. Marcin Baranski et al., "Higher Antioxidant and Lower Cadmium Concentrations and Lower Incidence of Pesticide Residues in Organically Grown Crops: A Systematic Literature Review and Meta-Analyses," British Journal of Nutrition 112, no. 5 (September 2014): 794–811, https://doi.org/10.1017/S0007114514001366.
51. Amir Sharon, Ziva Amsellem, and Jonathan Gressel, "Glyphosate Suppression of an Elicited Defense Response," Plant Physiology 98 (1992): 654–59, https://www.ncbi.nlm.nih.gov/pmc/articles/PMC1080240/pdf/plntphys00701-0254.pdf.
52. Mark L. Heiman and Frank L. Greenway, "A Healthy Gastrointestinal Microbiome Is Dependent on Dietary Diversity," Molecular Metabolism 5, no. 5 (May 2016): 317–20, doi:10.1016/j.molmet.2016.02.005.
53. Mesnage et al., "Integrated Multi-omics Analysis of the NK603 Roundup-Tolerant GM Maize" (see n. 31).
54. Mailin Gaupp-Berghausen et al., "Glyphosate-Based Herbicides Reduce the Activity and Reproduction of Earthworms and Lead to Increased Soil Nutrient Concentrations," Scientific Reports 5 (2015): 12886, doi:10.1038/srep12886.
55. Ib Borup Pedersen, "Changing from GMO to Non-GMO Natural Soy, Experiences from Denmark," Science in Society Archive, posted July 2014, accessed July 5, 2016, http://www.i-sis.org.uk/Changing_from_GMO_to_non-GMO_soy.php.
56. Henning Gerlach et al., "Oral Application of Charcoal and Humic Acids to Dairy Cows Influences Clostridium botulinum Blood Serum Antibody Level and Glyphosate Excretion in Urine," Journal of Clinical Toxicology 4 (2014): 186, doi:10.4172/2161-0495.1000186.
57. We realize that human and bovine digestive systems are not equivalent. In fact, however, one can buy supplements of humic acids to counteract the toxic effects of glyphosate already.
58. Monica Kruger et al., "Detection of Glyphosate Residues in Animals and Humans," Journal of Environmental and Analytical Toxicology 4, no. 2 (2014): 210–15, doi:10.4172/2161-0525.1000210.
59. Organophosphorous pesticides include insecticides that work as nerve agents, inhibiting the enzyme acetylcholinesterase needed for the production of

neurotransmitters. Lu Chensheng et al., "Organic Diets Significantly Lower Children's Dietary Exposure to Organophosphorus Pesticides," Environmental Health Perspectives 114, no. 2 (February 2006): 260–63, doi:10.1289/ehp.8418. See also, on children fed an exclusively organic diet will clear pesticides within a few days: Asa Bradman et al., "Effect of Organic Diet Intervention on Pesticide Exposures in Young Children Living in Low-Income Urban and Agricultural Communities," Environmental Health Perspectives 123, no. 10 (October 2015): 1086–93, doi:10.1289/ehp.1408660.

60. Landrigan and Benbrook, "GMOs, Herbicides, and Public Health" (see chap. 4 n. 27). We also note that at least one researcher from the food sciences and environment/ecology fields has been attacked for publishing research that shows GM crops are not self-contained—that is, that they spread to other crops accidentally. See the story of Ignacio Chapela, by John Ross, for instance, "The Sad Saga of Ignacio Chapela" Anderson Valley Advertiser, February 18, 2004, accessed October 15, 2016, http://www.theava.com/04/0218-chapela.html.
61. Dana Loomis et al., "Carcinogenicity of Lindane, DDT, and 2,4-Dichorophenoxyacetic Acid," The Lancet: Oncology 16, no. 8 (August 2015): 891–92, doi:10.1016/s1470-2045(15)00081-9.
62. They write: "In a 3-generation study, dicamba did not affect the reproductive capacity of rats. When rabbits were given doses of 0, 0.5, 1, 3, 10, or 20 (mg/kg)/day of technical dicamba from days 6 through 18 of pregnancy, toxic effects on the mothers, slightly reduced fetal body weights, and increased loss of fetuses occurred at the 10 mg/kg dose. The US Environmental Protection Agency has set the NOAEL for this study at 3 (mg/kg)/day." "Dicamba," Extension Toxicology Network, posted September 1993, accessed October 14, 2016, http://pmep.cce.cornell.edu/profiles/extoxnet/carbaryl-dicrotophos/dicamba-ext.html. See also: Caroline Cox, "Dicamba," Journal of Pesticide Reform 14, no. 1 (Spring 1994): 30–35, accessed June 8, 2017, http://www.panna.org/sites/default/files/dicamba-NCAP.pdf.
63. "Monsanto and DuPont Sign Dicamba Supply Agreement," Business Wire, posted July 7, 2016, http://www.businesswire.com/news/home/20160707005223/en/Monsanto-DuPont-Sign-Dicamba-Supply-Agreement.
64. Laura N. Vandenberg et al., "Hormones and Endocrine-Disrupting Chemicals: Low-Dose Effects and Nonmonotonic Dose Responses," Endocrine Reviews 33, no. 3 (June 2012): 378–455, doi:10.1210/er.2011-1050.
65. Mesnage et al., "Ethoxylated Adjuvants of Glyphosate-Based Herbicides" (see n. 31). This principle has been confirmed by experiments in living mammals. An in vivo study in pigs showed that the adjuvant POEA and commercial glyphosate herbicide formulations were toxic and lethal to the pigs, whereas glyphosate alone had no such effects. H.-L. Lee et al., "Comparative Effects of the Formulation

of Glyphosate-Surfactant Herbicides on Hemodynamics in Swine," Clinical Toxicology 47, no. 7 (August 2009): 651–58, doi:10.1080/15563650903158862. An in vivo study in rats showed that POEA and Roundup formulations containing POEA were more toxic than glyphosate alone. A. Adam et al., "The Oral and Intratracheal Toxicities of ROUNDUP and Its Components to Rats," Veterinary and Human Toxicology 39, no. 3 (June 1997): 147–51.

66. See Ashley Lukens's YouTube report: "Pesticides in Paradise: Our Keiki and 'Aina at Risk," 58:6, from Hawaii Center for Food Safety, posted by "centerforfoodsafety," December 3, 2015, accessed June 8, 2017, https://www.youtube.com/watch?v=0XEVQqlAXCY.
67. For a start, there is concern about the effect of organophosphate pesticides (not the same as glyphosate) on human oral microbiomes, see: "Pesticide Exposures Can Cause Changes in Oral Microbiome," American Society for Microbiology, posted November 11, 2016, accessed April 17, 2017, https://www.asm.org/index.php/journal-press-releases/94723-pesticide-exposures-can-cause-changes-in-oral-microbiome.

Chapter Fourteen: Can Autism Spectrum Disorder Be Improved by Way of Gut Health?

1. The vaccine/autism controversy has been another area in which the public trust has been eroded.
2. For these numbers see: http://www.cdc.gov/ncbddd/autism/data.html (accessed July 7, 2016). A useful reference for autism and environmental causes is the newsfeed for the Collaborative on Health and the Environment: http://www.healthandenvironment.org/autism (accessed July 25, 2017).
3. Claudia B. Avella-Garcia et al., "Acetaminophen Use in Pregnancy and Neurodevelopment: Attention Function and Autism Spectrum Symptoms," International Journal of Epidemiology 45, no. 6 (June 2016): 1987–96, doi:10.1093/ije/dyw115. See also the public version: Oxford University Press, "Prenatal Exposure to Acetaminophen May Increase Autism Spectrum and Hyperactivity Symptoms in Children," Science Daily, posted July 1, 2016, accessed June 9, 2017, http://www.sciencedaily.com/releases/2016/07/160701095445.htm.
4. D. Q. Ma et al., "Identification of Significant Association and Gene-Gene Interaction of GABA Receptor Subunit Genes in Autism," American Journal of Human Genetics 77, no. 3 (September 2005): 377–88, doi:10.1086/433195.
5. D. A. Rossignol, S. J. Genuis, and R. E. Frye, "Environmental Toxicants and Autism Spectrum Disorders: A Systematic Review," Translational Psychiatry 4 (2014): e360, doi:10.1038/tp.2014.4.
6. Jennifer G. Mulle, William G. Sharp, and Joseph F. Cubells, "The Gut Microbiome: A New Frontier in Autism Research," Current Psychiatry Reports 15,

no. 2 (February 2013): 337, doi:10.1007/s11920-012-0337-0; Shelly A. Buffington et al., "Microbial Reconstitution Reverses Maternal Diet-Induced Social and Synaptic Deficits in Offspring," Cell 165, no. 7 (June 16, 2016): 1762–75, doi:10.1016/j.cell.2016.06.001. For a lay summary, see research of Mauro Costa-Mattioli, "Microbes and Autism: Gut Feelings," The Economist, June 18, 2016, accessed June 9, 2017, http://www.economist.com/node/21700622.

7. Houston Methodist, "Autism Four Times Likelier When Mother's Thyroid Is Weakened," Science Daily, August 13, 2013, accessed June 9, 2017, https://www.sciencedaily.com/releases/2013/08/130813111730.htm.
8. Yehuda Shoenfeld, Nancy Agmon-Levin, and Lucija Tomljenovic, eds., Vaccines and Autoimmunity (Hoboken, NJ: John Wiley & Sons, 2015): 2–3. There is specific research on the possibility that neuroinflammation is linked to autism: Carlos A. Pardo-Villamizar, "Can Neuroinflammation Influence the Development of Autism Spectrum Disorders?" chap. 15 in Andrew Zimmerman, Autism: Current Theories and Evidence (Totowa, NJ: Humana Press, 2008), ebook.
9. Theoharis C. Theoharides, Shahrzad Asadi, and Arti B. Patel, "Focal Brain Inflammation and Autism," Journal of Neuroinflammation 10 (2013): 815, doi:10.1186/1742-2094-10-46.

Chapter Seventeen: Evidence-Based Medicine and Ecosystem Health

1. Izet Masic, Milan Miokovix, and Belma Muhamedagic, "Evidence Based Medicine—New Approaches and Challenges," Acta Informatica Medica 16, no. 4 (2008): 219–25, doi:10.5455/aim.2008.16.219-225.
2. Latham describes it as a kind of genetic engineering of the culture. Jonathan Latham, "Science and Social Control: Political Paralysis and the Genetics Agenda," Independent Science News, posted August 3, 2013, accessed June 9, 2017, https://www.independentsciencenews.org/science-media/science-and-social-control-political-paralysis-and-the-genetics-agenda. Also, this article published with Allison Wilson, "The Great DNA Data Deficit: Are Genes for Disease a Mirage?" Independent Science News, December 8, 2010, accessed June 9, 2017, https://www.independentsciencenews.org/health/the-great-dna-data-deficit.
3. Andrew Kimbrell, email message to Perro and Adams, July 20, 2016.
4. Joel Edwards, "Doctors against GMOs—Hear from Those Who Have Done the Research," Organic Lifestyle Magazine, August 2, 2015, accessed June 9, 2017, http://www.organiclifestylemagazine.com/doctors-against-gmos-hear-from-those-who-have-done-the-research.

INDEX

2,4-D (dichlorophenoxyacetic acid), 151, 152

abdominal pain
  Carlos case study, 115–19
  frequency of, 223n1
  Juan case study, 75–76, 78
  Quentin case study, 90–91
  Stephan case study, 91
acceptable levels concept, 112
acetylcholine, 40, 217n10
activist mothers, 203–8
"acute on chronic" disease, 19
additives
  FDA regulation of, 44–45
  GM technologies in, 102
  in processed foods, 36, 70
ADHD. *See* attention-deficit/hyperactivity disorder (ADHD)
ADIs (allowable daily intake levels), 140
adjuvants, pesticidal
  in combination pesticides, 153
  in glyphosate, 143, 145–46
  harms from, 153, 242–43n65
agrochemical industry
  attempts to ensure safety of chemicals, 38–39, 41
  discrediting of GM critics, 130–36
  ecosystems perspective on, 198–99
  glyphosate safety claims, 137, 138–39, 147
  GM food safety claims, 103, 112–13
  GM technology development, 43, 122–23
  profitability of, 199
  sponsorship of food safety research, 32, 46, 47, 133
agroecology, 125–26
allergies
  gut microbiome connection, 67, 75
  increase in, 7
  off-target gene effects and, 129
  Stephanie case study, 186–87
  See also food allergies
Alliance for Science, 123
allostatic loads, 83
allowable daily intake levels (ADIs), 140
Altered Genes, Twisted Truth (Druker), 44–45, 129–130
American Academy of Environmental Medicine, 201
American Academy of Pediatrics, 156
American Medical Association (AMA), 26, 191, 193, 194
American Microbiome Institute, 59
Amish people, 94, 226n3
AMPA, 143, 145, 236nn8, 9
animal research
  Bt toxin crops, 143–44
  glyphosate, 142–48
  GM foods, 21, 108–9, 112, 130–36
  health benefits from elimination of GM foods, 150–51
  relationship between microbiome and health, 65, 66
antibiotic resistance, 70
antibiotics
  dysbiosis associated with, 69–70
  in food production, 69–70
  glyphosate as, 73, 105, 144, 227n9
  role in leaky gut, 89
  Trevor case study, 11, 12, 15, 65
  Willa case study, 2–3
antioxidants
  epigenetic qualities, 72
  in organic food, 126
  Zoe case study, 97
Antoniou, Michael, 142, 144, 146, 147
apples, genetically modified, 102, 128–29
Arrieta, Marie-Claire, 66
asthma
  benefits of childhood exposure to microbes, 94
  increase in, x
  Irene case study, 6
atrazine, 40
attention-deficit/hyperactivity disorder (ADHD)

attention-deficit/hyperactivity disorder (*continued*)
  increase in, x
  reliance on pharmaceutical solutions, 158, 160
autism spectrum disorder, 169–177
  benefits of improving gut health, 169, 176–77
  Carlos case study, 115–19
  debate over causes of, 174–76
  increase in, x, 175
  Sami case study, 170–74, 177, 181
autoimmune disorders
  diplomatic metaphor for healing, 82, 83
  rise in, 82, 88–90, 225n3
  role of gut health in, 66–67, 75, 85–86, 225n7
  See also specific disorders

Bacillus thuringiensis (Bt) toxin crops. *See* Bt (*Bacillus thuringiensis*) toxin crops
bacteria
  in the microbiome, 59, 60
  oversanitization concerns, 94–95
  ratio with human cells, 60
  See also microbiome; *specific types*
Bartonella infections, 188
Bayer Pharmaceuticals, 199
behavior problems
  Carlos case study, 115–16
  connection to chronic pesticides exposure, 95–98
  Mike case study, 159–168
  reliance on pharmaceutical solutions, 158
  Sami case study, 170–74
  Zoe case study, 95–98
  See also autism spectrum disorder
Berkowitz, Lindsay, 216n1
Bifidobacteria, 69, 72, 98, 117
bioaccumulation of toxicants
  ease of, 42
  glyphosate, 139, 140, 235–36nn8, 9
  lack of research on, 46
biotechnology, 38–39
  See also genetic modification (GM) technologies
birth defects, association with pesticides, 40, 133
birth process, effect on newborn's microbiome, 61, 64–65
Blair, Tony, 132
Blaser, Martin, 67, 94
blood-brain barrier, 146, 181
book resources, 211
brain problems. *See* neurocognitive problems
breast milk, glyphosate found in, 140, 141
Brillat-Savarin, Jean, 11
Brown, Gabe, 126
Bt (*Bacillus thuringiensis*) toxin crops
  animal research on, 143–44
  conflicting evidence of equivalence of, 110, 228–29n18
  loss of selectivity, 107
  overlap with Roundup Ready crops, 48, 107
  reasons to be concerned about, 103–4, 106–7, 110
  regulation of, 112
  resistance to, 152–53
B vitamin supplements, 88, 97, 171, 173, 206

Caesarean sections, 64–65
call to action, 203–8
Cani, Patrice, 70
Carlos (case study), 115–19
Carman, Judy, 143–44, 239n36
Carnegie Foundation, 26
Caroline (case study), 90–91
Carrasco, Andres, 133–34
Carrie (case study), 50–52, 55
Carson, Rachel, xii, 37, 112, 199
case studies
  Carlos (autism), 115–19
  Caroline (celiac disease), 90–91
  Carrie (respiratory problems), 50–52, 55
  debate over validity of, 192–93
  Ernesto (kidney problems), 117–18
  Helen (eczema), 204–7
  Irene (asthma), 6
  Jason (appetite problems), 52, 53–55
  Juan (gastrointestinal problems), 75–80
  Kayla (developmental delay), 178–180, 181
  Marilyn (Sjogren's disorder), 50–56
  Mike (behavioral problems), 159–168
  Quentin (abdominal pain and failure to thrive), 90–91
  Sami (autism), 170–74, 177, 181
  Sean (eczema and food sensitivities), 4–6, 16
  Stephan (gluten sensitivity), 91

Stephanie (neurocognitive problems), 183, 184–89
Sylvie (eczema), 204–7
Trevor (ulcerative colitis), 11–15, 27, 32, 65
Willa (GERD), 1–3, 16
Zoe (behavior problems), 95–98
celiac disease
Caroline case study, 90–91
increase in, x
mechanisms of, 85–87
Quentin case study, 90–91
Stephanie case study, 187–88
See also gluten sensitivity
Center for Child and Adolescent Health Policy, 7
Chapela, Ignacio, 242n60
Charge Study (UC Davis), 40
chemical toxicants. *See* toxicants
child development
benefits of exposure to microbes, 66, 94
establishment of healthy gut, 61–66
global developmental delay, 177, 178–180, 181
pesticide-associated neurodevelopmental concerns, 40, 146
chlorpyrifos, 40, 218–19n24
chromosomal abnormalities, 179–180
chronic health concerns
"acute on chronic" disease, 19
common underlying causes of, xi
difficulty in diagnosing and treating, x–xi, 19, 193, 200
increase in, ix–x, 7
pharmaceutical vs. food-focused solutions, 27–28
role of gut health in, 24, 66–69
See also specific conditions
chronic reference dose levels (cRfDs), 47, 141
cilia, 68, 84
cleaning products, toxicity of, 94
clinical guidelines
gap with new research, 191–95
lack of awareness of food concerns, 28, 32, 33
need for, in food-focused integrative medicine, 198, 208
clinical trials
for GM technologies, 111
lack of, for food-focused integrative medicine, 193, 194
clinicians, food-focused, 34
Clinton, Bill, 132
Clostridium difficile infections, 67
COEH (Council on Environmental Health), 156
cognitive problems. *See* neurocognitive problems
colitis
increase in, x
Trevor case study, 11–15, 27, 32, 65
Columbia University Medical Center, 86–87
combat metaphor for immune system, 81–82, 224n3
combination pesticides, presumed safety of, 152–53
commensalism, 63
See also symbiosis
comorbidities, 183–190
complexity of, 183–84, 200
Stephanie case study, 183, 184–89
systems perspective approach to health, 189–190, 200
compositional profiling, 113
constipation
Carlos case study, 116
Kayla case study, 178, 180
pharmaceutical vs. food-focused solutions, 27
Sami case study, 171, 173
Zoe case study, 96
conventional medicine
difficulties with chronic diseases, x–xi, 19, 193, 200
history of scientific medicine, 26–31
lack of awareness of food concerns, 17, 31–34
limitations of, 3–6, 7, 16–18
need for new model, 198, 200–202
reliance on pharmaceutical and biotechnological solutions, 18, 23–24, 25, 198–99
corn, genetically modified
animal research on, 132–33, 146
glyphosate- and 2,4-D-resistant, 151
Séralini, Gilles-Eric research on, 143
Xtend system, 152
cotton, genetically modified, 48, 102, 103, 151
Council on Environmental Health (COEH), 156
cRfDs (chronic reference dose levels), 47, 141

CRISPR technologies, 128
croup, 20
Cry protein, 106, 133

dairy-free diet
  Carlos case study, 117
  Carrie case study, 55
  Juan case study, 77–78
  Marilyn case study, 53
  Sami case study, 173
  Sean case study, 5, 6
  Sylvie case study, 205
  Trevor case study, 13, 14
  Willa case study, 3
  Zoe case study, 97
DAN (Defeat Autism Now), 171, 172–73
David, Lawrence, 68
Daytrana, 160
DDT, xii, 37
Defeat Autism Now (DAN), 171, 172–73
deregulated status of crops, 111, 112, 128–29
desiccant and ripening agent use of glyphosate, 106, 138
detoxification
  Carlos case study, 116–17
  Helen case study, 205
  Mike case study, 162, 164
  Sami case study, 171, 173–74
  Sylvie case study, 205, 206
  Zoe case study, 97–98
diarrhea
  Helen case study, 205–7
  in pigs on GM feed, 150
dicamba, 152, 242n62
diet
  difficulty of changing, 33
  in systems perspective approach to health, 189–190
  therapeutic possibilities of, 56, 61
  See also food; *specific case studies*
digestion, 72, 84
digestive disorders. *See* gastrointestinal problems
diplomatic metaphor for microbiome, 82–83
dizziness, Stephanie case study, 184–89
DNA methylation, 72
  See also epigenetics
double-stranded RNA (dsRNA), 128, 152–53
Druker, Steven, 44–45, 112, 129–130
dry eyes and mouth, 52, 53
dysbiosis
  Carlos case study, 116, 117
  causes of, 69–71
  defined, 64
  glyphosate contribution to, 149
  increasing research on, 30, 65, 66
  Juan case study, 75–80
  Mike case study, 159–168
  relationship with diseases, 24, 66–69, 88–90, 180–82
  role in gluten sensitivity, 87–88
  uncommon diagnosis of, 80
  See also leaky gut

ear infections
  Carrie case study, 50–51
  Willa case study, 2–3
E. coli infections, 11, 12
ecomedicine concept, 196
ecosystems approach
  need for, 58, 196–98
  rethinking of food and pharmaceutical systems, 198–202
eczema and atopic dermatitis
  increase in, x
  Sean case study, 4–6, 16
  Sylvie case study, 204–7
edible foodlike substances, as term, 7–8, 36
egg sensitivities, 5
Eisenberg, David, 28
endocrine disorders, 40, 89–90, 142
enhanced GM foods, 102, 123, 125, 127–28
Enlist Duo herbicide, 151
enteric nervous system, 169
environmental exposure to toxicants
  frequency of, 41–42
  overview, 93–95
  role in increasing chronic health concerns, 7, 9
  well-informed futility, 93, 98–100
  Zoe case study, 95–98
Environmental Health (journal), 142
Environmental Pollutants Profile urine test, 96, 116
EPA. *See* US Environmental Protection Agency (EPA)

Index

epigenetics
  defined, 72
  interaction with gut microbiome, 72, 73
  Marilyn case study, 56
epithelial layer, 84, 85
equivalence criterion
  Bt crops, 110, 228–29n18
  critiques of GM food studies, 108, 110
  focus on, 46
  presumed safety of GM foods, 155
  reliance on industry claims, 103, 111–12, 113, 230n25
Ernesto (case study), 117–18
Eskenazi, Brenda, 39–41, 217n10
evidence-based medicine, 191–202
  ecosystem health importance, 196–98
  food health importance, 195–96
  gap between clinical guidelines and new research, 191–95
  rethinking of food and pharmaceutical systems, 198–202

failure to thrive
  Jason case study, 52, 53–55
  Quentin case study, 90–91
farmworkers, exposure to pesticides, 40–41
Fasano, Alessio, 85–86, 225n7
fat, chemicals stored in, 42
FDA. *See* US Food and Drug Administration (FDA)
fecal transplants, 67
fiber, importance to gut health, 68, 85, 88
film resources, 212
Finlay, B. Brett, 66, 94
firmicutes, 68
five Rs (remove, replace, reinoculate, repair, and rebalance), 74, 79
Flavr Savr tomato, 101
Flexner Report, 26
FluMist, 186–87, 189
food
  conventional medicine lack of focus on, 31–34
  as information for the microbiome, 71–73
  lack of research on, 30
  role of hidden ingredients, 33
  See also diet; genetically modified (GM) food; organic food
food additives. *See* additives
food allergies
  Carrie case study, 51
  immune response tests for, 74
  increase in, ix–x, 7, 33
  intolerances and sensitivities vs., 5, 77
  See also food sensitivities
Food and Agricultural Organization, 140
Food and Chemical Toxicology (journal), 133
Food and Nutrition Board, 70
food-focused clinicians, 34
food-focused integrative medicine
  benefits of, xvi–xvii, 9–10
  conflicting scientific claims, 23–24, 130
  ecomedicine concept, 196
  evidence for, 193–94
  food as medicine, 15–18
  need for clinical guidelines, 198
  overview, 24–25
food immune response tests, 74, 76–77, 78
food intolerances, 77
  See also food allergies; food sensitivities
food pyramids, 25
food security argument for GM foods, 122, 124, 125–26, 128
food sensitivities
  allergies and intolerances vs., 5, 77
  Carlos case study, 116
  Carrie case study, 51, 52, 55
  connection to nonorganic foods, 52
  difficulty diagnosing, 59
  immune response tests for, 74
  increase in, 7
  Juan case study, 76–77
  Kayla case study, 178–79
  Marilyn case study, 51
  Mike case study, 162–64, 166
  Sean case study, 5
  See also food allergies; *specific types*
Friends of the Earth, 129, 140
functional medicine, 74, 79
funding for research. *See* research funding

Gaia hypothesis, 63
Galanthus nivalis agglutinin (GNA), 131, 132
gastrointestinal problems
  frequency of, 223n1
  reliance on pharmaceutical solutions, 24, 25, 27–28

gastrointestinal problems (*continued*)
  rise in, 88–90
  See also specific conditions
gastrointestinal reflux disease (GERD), x, 1–3, 16
gene editing technologies, 114, 128–29, 230n28
generally recognized as safe (GRAS) status, 44–45, 112
gene-silencing technology, 128
genetically modified (GM) food, 120–136
  animal research on, 21, 108–9, 112, 130–36
  arguments in support of, 122–24
  bans on, 114, 231n29
  benefits of elimination of, 150–51
  critiques of studies suggesting safety of, 108–9, 110
  debate over safety of, xii–xiii, xv, xvi, 120–22, 124–130
  difficulty of separating effects of pesticides, 143
  enhanced, 102, 123, 125, 127–28
  generally recognized as safe (GRAS) status, 44–45, 112
  history of, 101–3
  increase in consumption of, xii
  lack of research on, 71
  molecular compositional profiling, 113
  presumed safety of, 155
  support for labeling of, 114, 121
  ubiquity across socioeconomic levels, 57
  Xtend system, 152
Genetic Literacy Project, 123
genetic modification (GM) technologies
  agrochemicals associated with, 43
  benefits of, 103
  crops of concern, 48–49
  development of, 38–39
  ecosystems perspective on, 198–99
  history of, 101–3
  medical applications, 111
  off-target effects, 129
  reasons to be concerned about, 48–49, 100, 103, 135–36
  role in pesticide resistance, 39
  testing on humans, 111
German Biological Medicines, 78, 224n3
gliadin, 85
global developmental delay, 177, 178–180, 181
glutathione supplements, 97
gluten, 70, 85, 86
gluten-free diet
  Carlos case study, 117
  conventional vs. integrative medicine views, 219–220n2
  Juan case study, 77–78
  Marilyn case study, 53, 55
  Quentin case study, 90
  Sami case study, 173
  Sean case study, 5
  Stephan case study, 91
  Stephanie case study, 187–88
  Sylvie case study, 205, 207
  Trevor case study, 13, 14
  Willa case study, 3
  Zoe case study, 97
glutenin, 85
gluten sensitivity
  Carlos case study, 116
  connection to Sjogren's disorder, 55, 219–220n2
  Marilyn case study, 53, 55
  mechanisms of, 86–88
  Sean case study, 5
  Stephan case study, 91
  See also celiac disease
glyphosate (Roundup), 137–156
  adjuvants to, 143, 145–46
  allowed levels of, 138–39, 140–42, 235–36nn8, 9, 238n23
  antibiotic formulation, 73, 105, 144, 227n9
  chelating aspects, 145, 149
  in combination with other pesticides, 151–54
  dangers of exposure to, 40
  desiccant and ripening agent use of, 106, 138
  effects on children, 154–56
  elimination of GM foods from diet, 150–51
  identification as probable carcinogen, 147
  impact on nutritional quality of food, 148–49, 241n49
  industry claims of safety, 137
  inert ingredients, concerns about, 145
  mechanisms of, 104–5
  as organophosphate pesticide, 217n10
  persistence of, 139–140
  research on, 133–34, 142–48
  resistance to, 151–54

rise in use of, 138
ubiquity in human bodies, 138–142
GM. *See* genetically modified (GM) food; genetic modification (GM) technologies
GM Freeze, 140
GMO Answers website, 227n9
GMO Myths and Truths (Robinson et al.), 129
GM Watch, 234n32, 235n6
GNA (*Galanthus nivalis* agglutinin), 131, 132
golden rice, 127, 232n14
Goodall, Jane, 35, 43
The Good Gut (Sonnenburg and Sonnenburg), 68
Greenpeace, 230n21, 232n14
green pharmacy approach, 30, 196
Greer, Beth, 42
Gulp: Adventures on the Alimentary Canal (Roach), 62
gut health
diagnostic tests for, 21, 74–75, 80
diplomatic metaphor for, 82–83
health benefits from elimination of GM foods, 150–51
importance for pharmaceutical therapies, 158–59
need for personalized approach, 181, 184
possible connection to autism, 171, 177
role in chronic conditions, 24
See also leaky gut
gut microbiome, 59–73
alterable nature of, 61
antibiotic effects on, 69–70, 89, 144
defined, 60
diplomatic metaphor for, 82–83
foods affecting, 67–68
glyphosate effects on, 144–48
importance to health, 24, 61–62, 66–69
increasing research on, 30, 59–62
information from food and, 71–73
nutrients produced by, 72
resiliency of, 67–68
role in digestion, 72
variability in, 71
See also dysbiosis; symbiosis

Hahnemann, Samuel, 17, 215n1
Haraway, Donna, 83
headaches
increase in, x
Stephanie case study, 185, 187, 188
See also migraines
Helen (case study), 204–7
Helicobacter pylori, 67
Hippocrates, 17
histone modification, 72
See also epigenetics
HLA (human leukocyte antigen) markers, 85
Hogan, Simon, 234n38
homeopathics
Carlos case study, 117
for croup, 20
Jason case study, 54
Juan case study, 77–78
Kayla case study, 179, 180
Marilyn case study, 55
Mike case study, 162
overview, 215n1
Quentin case study, 90
role in integrative medicine, 17
Sami case study, 173
Sean case study, 5
Stephanie case study, 187, 188
Sylvie case study, 205
Trevor case study, 15
Willa case study, 3
Honeycutt, Zen, 199, 235n38
Huber, Don, 137
human leukocyte antigen (HLA) markers, 85
human studies
costs of, 194
on glyphosate levels, 139–140, 141, 146
lack of, for GM foods, 110, 111–12, 125, 154–56
on medical GM technologies, 103, 111
need for, 144–46, 155–56
humic acids, 150, 241n57
hygiene hypothesis, 94

IARC (International Agency for Research on Cancer), 147
IBS (irritable bowel syndrome), x, 68
IgA immune reactions, 5, 74, 76–77, 223–24n2
IgE immune reactions, 5, 77
IgG immune reactions, 5, 74, 76–77, 223–24n2
immune responses
to gluten, 86, 87
from leaky gut, 89

immune responses (*continued*)
possible connection to autism, 175–76
Sean case study, 5
immune response tests, 74, 77, 223–24n2
immune system
combat metaphor for, 81–82, 224n3
role of gut health in, 62, 66–67
immunizations, controversy over possible link to autism, 115, 170, 174–75
In Defense of Food (Pollan), 7–8
industrial food
defined, xii, 101
ecosystems perspective on, 197–98
potential role in chronic health concerns, xii–xvi
rethinking of, 198–202, 208
toxicants in, 8–10, 35–37, 43
See also genetically modified (GM) food
inert ingredients. *See* adjuvants, pesticidal
infant mortality, 213n1
Innate potato, 102, 128
Institute for Responsible Technology, 227n6
Institute of Medicine, 70
integrative medicine
emergence of field, 29–30, 216n1
lack of focus on food, 29–30
turn to, 3–6
See also food-focused integrative medicine
International Agency for Research on Cancer (IARC), 147
International Assessment of Agricultural Knowledge, Science, and Technology for Development report, 125–26
International Rice Research Institute (IRRI), 232n14
intestinal permeability. *See* leaky gut
Irene (case study), 6
IRRI (International Rice Research Institute), 232n14
irritable bowel syndrome (IBS), x, 68

Jason (case study), 52, 53–55
Juan (case study), 75–80

Kayla (case study), 178–180, 181
Kennedy, Robert F., Jr., 199
Kessler, David, 36
kidney disorders
Ernesto case study, 117–18
from glyphosate, 142, 146
in rats fed GM corn, 132–33
Kimbrell, Andrew, 197

Lactobacilli spp.
Carlos case study, 117
in probiotics, 69
role in gut health, 175
Zoe case study, 98
LaDuke, Winona, 199
Lappe, Frances Moore, 199
Larry, Pamm, 199
Latham, Jonathan, 195
leaky gut
Carlos case study, 116, 117
causes of, 85
comorbidities as both cause and effect of, 183–84
connection to neurocognitive problems, 181–82
defined, 85
effects of toxicants in food, 89, 91–92
glyphosate contribution to, 149
Mike case study, 159–168
in pests, from Bt toxin, 106, 107
possible connection to autism, 174–76
recent research on, 83–88
role in gluten sensitivity, 87–88
learned helplessness, 99, 100
lectins, research on, 130–31
Let Them Eat Dirt (Finlay and Arrieta), 66
lipopolysaccharides, 89
liver problems
from glyphosate, 142, 146–47
increase in, 57
in rats fed GM corn, 132–33

MADLs (maximum allowable dose levels), 47
magic bullet medicine, as term, 27
mainstream medicine. *See* conventional medicine
Malkan, Stacy, 199
Margulis, Lynn, 63, 83
Marilyn (case study), 50–56
Martin, Emily, 81–82, 224n3
Martineau, Belinda, 113, 234n38
Masic, Izet, 191

Index

maximum allowable dose levels (MADLs), 47
maximum residue levels (MRLs), 139
mental disorders
  increase in, x
  Jason case study, 54
  Mike case study, 159–168
  See also neurocognitive problems
mercury toxicity, 170
metabolomics, 108, 109, 142
methylation deficiency
  Carlos case study, 116
  Kayla case study, 180
  Sylvie case study, 206
  Zoe case study, 97
microbiome
  alterable nature of, 61
  defined, 60
  diplomatic metaphor for, 82–83
  establishment during early childhood, 61–66, 94
  hygiene hypothesis and, 94
  importance of nurturing, 83
  increasing research on, 30–31
  shikimate pathway in bacteria of, 105
  See also gut microbiome
migraines
  increase in, x
  pharmaceutical vs. food-focused solutions, 27
  Stephanie case study, 186, 188
  See also headaches
Mike (case study), 159–168
military metaphor for immune system, 81–82, 224n3
milk, from cows treated with rBGH, 102, 226–27n5
  See also dairy-free diet
Miller, Daphne, 199
Missing Microbes (Blaser), 67
modern industrial food. *See* industrial food
molecular compositional profiling, 113
Monsanto Corporation, 38, 104–5, 132, 199
movie resources, 212
Mozaffarian, Dariush, 23
MRLs (maximum residue levels), 139
MTHFR (methyltetrahydrofolate reductase enzyme) status test
  Carlos case study, 116
  Kayla case study, 180
  Zoe case study, 97
mucosal layer, 68, 85
Mundipur, 78
mushrooms, genetically modified, 129
mutualism, 63
  See also symbiosis
mycobiome, defined, 60

NAC (N-acetyl cysteine), 97
National Academies of Sciences, Engineering, and Medicine, 122, 123
National Cancer Institute, 42
National Center for Complementary and Integrative Health, 29
National Institutes of Health, 29
National Microbiome Initiative, 30
National Pesticide Information Center, 147
National Primary Drinking Water Regulations, 147
NCWS (non-celiac wheat sensitivity), 87
neurocognitive problems, 157–168
  complexity of, 157–59
  difficulty diagnosing, 157–59
  Kayla case study, 178–180, 181
  Mike case study, 159–168
  role of gut health in, 89–90, 178–182
  Stephanie case study, 184–89
  See also specific disorders
neurodevelopmental concerns
  from chronic exposure to pesticides, 40, 146
  global developmental delay, 177, 178–180, 181
neurotransmitter level tests, 74
NOAELs (no observed adverse effect levels), 46–47
non-celiac wheat sensitivity (NCWS), 87
no observed adverse effect levels (NOAELs), 46–47, 112
no significant risk levels (NSRLs), 47, 141, 147
nutrition
  conventional medicine lack of focus on, 31–34
  glyphosate effects on, 148–49
  medical school teachings on, 25, 31–32
  need for research on, 30, 34
  new research on, 25
  organic vs. GM crops, 125, 126, 148–49, 241n49

Obama, Barack, 40
obesity
  increase in, x
  links to gut microbial composition, 69
  Mike case study, 162, 167–68
O'Brien, Robyn, 199
off-target genetic engineering effects, 129
omega three and six fatty acid supplements, 98, 206
organic food
  Carlos case study, 117, 118–19
  Carrie case study, 51–52, 55
  ecosystems perspective on, 199
  Ernesto case study, 118–19
  importance of, 8
  Jason case study, 55
  Juan case study, 77–78
  Kayla case study, 179
  Marilyn case study, 55
  Mike case study, 165, 168
  need for support from science and medicine, 201
  for neurocognitive problems, 158
  nutrition of, vs. GM crops, 125, 126, 148–49, 241n49
  profitability of, 201–2
  Quentin case study, 90
  reduced risk of glyphosate exposure, 150–51
  Sami case study, 172, 173
  Stephan case study, 91
  Trevor case study, 14
  Willa case study, 3
  yields, vs. GM crops, 126
  Zoe case study, 97
organochlorines, 40
organophosphate pesticides, 40, 116, 151, 217n10, 231n30

Patton, Sharyle, 50
Pederson, Ib, 150
perfect storm concept, 6–8
Perkel, Jenny, 1
pesticide foods, 46, 49
pesticides
  absorption into plants, 41
  acute vs. chronic exposure to, 95
  adjuvants in, 143, 145–46, 153, 242–43n65
  attempt to reduce via GM foods, xii
  Carlos case study, 116
  combination, 152
  dangers of exposure to, 39–41
  difficulty of separating effects of GM foods, 143
  growing resistance of, 39
  increase in use of, 106, 151–54
  lack of research on, 71
  plants as, 106
  regulation of, 37–38, 45–49
  spraying of soil vs. crops, 48
  Zoe case study, 95–98
  See also specific types
pharmaceutical industry
  collaboration with AMA, 26
  research funding, 24
pharmaceutical solutions
  benefits of, 195–96
  ease of, 33
  green pharmacy approach, 30, 196
  magic bullet medicine, 27
  Mike case study, 160–62
  for neurocognitive problems, 158
  pill for ill medicine, as term, 19, 23, 195
  relationship with clinical medicine, 27
  reliance on, 18, 23–24, 25, 195–96
  rethinking of, 198–202
phenylalanine, 88, 105
phytoalexins, 149
pill for ill medicine, as term, 19, 23, 195
planetary patriotism, as term, 39
plant-incorporated protectants (PIPs), 45
POEA, 145, 236n9, 242–43n65
political change, need for, 207
Pollan, Michael, 7–8, 36, 63, 70, 199
polybrominated diphenyl ethers (PBDEs), 217–18n19
polymerase chain reaction (PCR) tests, 74, 76
potatoes, genetically modified, 102, 128–29, 130–32
pregnancy
  Bt toxin found in blood of pregnant women, 110
  chemicals found in blood of pregnant women, 42, 217–18n19
  dysbiosis during, 64
  establishment of healthy gut in fetus, 61–62, 64

glyphosate found in urine of pregnant women, 140, 146
probiotics
for antibiotics users, 69
Carlos case study, 117
Helen case study, 205
Jason case study, 54
Juan case study, 77–78
Kayla case study, 179
Mike case study, 162
Quentin case study, 91
Sami case study, 172
Stephanie case study, 188
Sylvie case study, 205, 206
Willa case study, 3
Zoe case study, 97–98
processed foods
additives in, 36, 70
questions about effect on gut health, 49
toxicants in, 35–36
proteomics, 142, 155
Pusztai, Arpad, 130–32, 146, 234n32
pyrethroids, 40

Quentin (case study), 90–91
quinolinates, 116
quorum sensing, 64

rBGH (bovine growth hormone), 102, 226–27n5
regulation
assumed safety of chemicals until proven otherwise, 45–46
conflicts of interest in, 114
debate over safety of GM foods, 110–15
difficulty of keeping up with technological advances, 154
of pesticides, 37–38, 45–49
as public good, 44–49
reliance on industry claims, 111–12, 113, 114
remove, replace, reinoculate, repair, and rebalance (five Rs), 74, 79
research
critiques of GM food studies, 108–9, 110
EPA use of, 46–47
on gut microbiome, 30, 59–62
on impact of glyphosate on health, 133–34, 142–48
on integrative approaches, 29–30
lack of, on food and nutrition, 30, 32, 33, 34
questions about reliability of, 32
support for GM technologies, 122–24
See also animal research; human studies
research funding
GM food studies, 109, 133, 134
reliance on pharmaceutical and biotechnological industries, 24, 194
resistance
to antibiotics, 70
due to GM technologies, 125
to glyphosate, 106
increased use of pesticides due to, 151–54
resources, 211–12
RNA interference (RNAi), 128, 152–53
Roach, Mary, 62
Roundup. *See* glyphosate (Roundup)
Roundup Ready crops
history of, 104–6
overlap with Bt crops, 107
reasons to be concerned about, 48, 103
Rowett Institute, 130, 132

salmon, genetically modified, 129
Sami (case study), 170–74, 177, 181
sancti-mommies, as term, 208
Schmeiser, Percy, 235n38
Schneiderman, Howard, 38–39
scientific medicine, history of, 26–31
Sean (case study), 4–6, 16
seeds
costs of GM seeds, 124
glyphosate- and 2,4-D-resistant, 151
patented, 103
treatment with insecticides, 107
vulnerabilities of GM monocultures, 124
Seneff, Stephanie, 234n38
Séralini, Gilles-Eric, 132–33, 142, 143, 146, 234n32
Shetterly, Caitlin, 199
shikimate pathway, 105, 139
Shiva, Vandana, 199
signaling molecules, 64
Silent Spring (Carson), xii, 37
Sjogren's disorder, 53, 55, 219–220n2
small intestine, 84–85, 89
Smith, Jeffrey, 199, 235n38

The Social Transformation of American Medicine (Starr), 27
soil, glyphosate effects on, 149
Soil Association, 139
Sonnenburg, Erica, 68
Sonnenburg, Justin, 68
soybeans, genetically modified
  animal research on, 143–44, 146
  glyphosate- and 2,4-D-resistant, 151
  introduction of, 101
  Xtend system, 152
soy-free diet
  Sami case study, 173
  Trevor case study, 13, 14
  Willa case study, 3
Spinning Food (report), 129
Starr, Paul, 26–27
Steingraber, Sandra, 36, 41, 93, 98–99, 100
Stephan (case study), 91
Stephanie (case study), 183, 184–89
steroids
  Sean case study, 4
  Trevor case study, 12–13, 15
stomachaches. *See* abdominal pain
Stone, Glenn Davis, 121
stool marker tests
  benefits of, 21, 74
  Juan case study, 76, 78
  Mike case study, 163
substantial equivalence criterion. *See* equivalence criterion
sugar-free diet
  Marilyn case study, 53
  Mike case study, 163–65, 166–68
  Trevor case study, 13, 14
supplements
  Carlos case study, 117
  Helen case study, 205
  Juan case study, 77–78
  Kayla case study, 180
  Sami case study, 171, 172
  Stephanie case study, 188
  Sylvie case study, 205, 206
  Zoe case study, 97, 98
Sustainable Pulse, 133
Swansburg, John, 81
Swanson, Nancy, 234n38
SyGest, 79
Sylvie (case study), 204–7
symbiosis
  as model for gut health, 82, 83, 200
  theory of, 62–66
systems perspective approach to health, 189–190, 200

Taubes, Gary, 36
tomatoes, genetically modified, 101
toxicants
  agrochemicals, 39–41, 42–44, 45–49, 112–15
  allostatic loads, 83
  bioaccumulation of, 42, 46, 139, 140, 235–36nn8, 9
  in cleaning products, 94
  excessive allostatic load of, 83
  from food, xi–xiii, 6, 7–9, 32–37, 43–44, 181–82
  from GM foods, 120, 130–36
  increased exposure to, xi–xii, 93–95
  naturally occurring, 223n38
  non-agricultural routes of exposure to, 41–42
  from off-target effects of GM technologies, 129
  purported safety of, 46–49
  role in leaky gut, 89, 91–92
  role of hidden ingredients, 33
  varying effects on different people, 57–58
  See also Bt (*Bacillus thuringiensis*) toxin crops; dysbiosis; glyphosate (Roundup); pesticides; *specific case studies*
toxic environment. *See* environmental exposure to toxicants
The Toxic Sandbox (Steingraber), 41
Toxic Substances Control Act (1976), 45
Trevor (case study), 11–15, 27, 32, 65
Trump, Donald, 40
tryptophan, 88, 105
Turnbaugh, Peter, 68–69, 219n2
tyrosine, 88, 105

ulcerative colitis. *See* colitis
Union of Concerned Scientists, 101
United Nations (UN), 125
University of Oregon, 147
urinary environmental pollutants profile, 96, 116
US Coordinated Framework on Biotechnology, 114

Index

US Department of Agriculture (USDA)
deregulated status of crops, 111, 112, 128–29
lack of adequate oversight of chemicals, 44, 45–48
regulation of GMOs, 112
US Environmental Protection Agency (EPA)
Enlist Duo approval, 151–52
glyphosate safety levels, 138, 147
lack of adequate oversight of chemicals, 40, 44, 45–47, 48, 219n24
little ability to regulate toxicants, 112–13
US Food and Drug Administration (FDA)
Campaign Against Nutritional Quackery, 26
lack of adequate oversight of chemicals, 44–45, 47–48
little ability to regulate GM technologies, 113
reliance on industry claims, 111–12
voluntary notification systems, 111–12

vaccinations, controversy over possible link to autism, 115, 170, 174–75
Velasquez-Manoff, Moises, 94
villi, 68, 84, 85, 86
virome, defined, 60
Vrain, Thierry, 234n38

warrior moms, 203–8
website resources, 212
Weibe, Gerhardt, 98–99
well-informed futility, 93, 98–100
wheat
genetically modified, 103, 227n8
non-celiac wheat sensitivity, 87
See also celiac disease; gluten-free diet
Willa (case study), 1–3, 16
Woodruff, Tracey, 42
World Bank, 125, 126
World Health Organization, 147, 235n8

Xtend system, 152

yields, organic vs. GM crops, 126

Zoe (case study), 95–98
zombie paradigm, as term, 197
zonulin, 84, 85–86, 89, 225n7

ABOUT THE AUTHORS

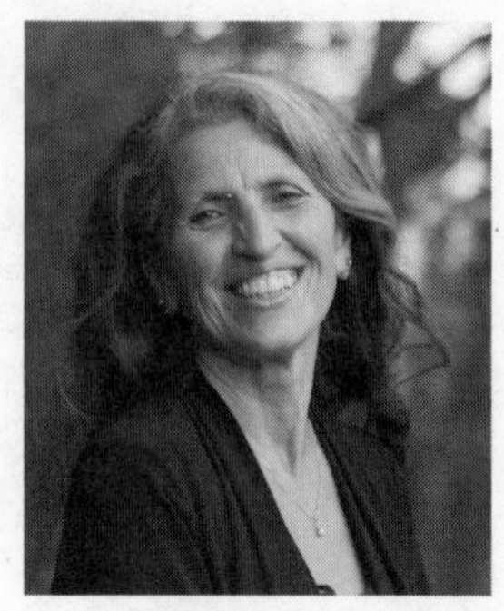
KYAWT THIRI NYUNT

Michelle Perro, MD, is a veteran pediatrician with over thirty-five years of experience in acute and integrative medicine. More than ten years ago, Dr. Perro transformed her clinical practice to include pesticide and health advocacy. She has both directed and worked as attending physician from New York's Metropolitan Hospital to UCSF Benioff Children's Hospital Oakland. Dr. Perro has managed her own business, Down to Earth Pediatrics, a holistic urgent care clinic for children. For the past four years, she has been an integrative physician at the Institute for Health and Healing, part of Sutter Pacific Medical Center.

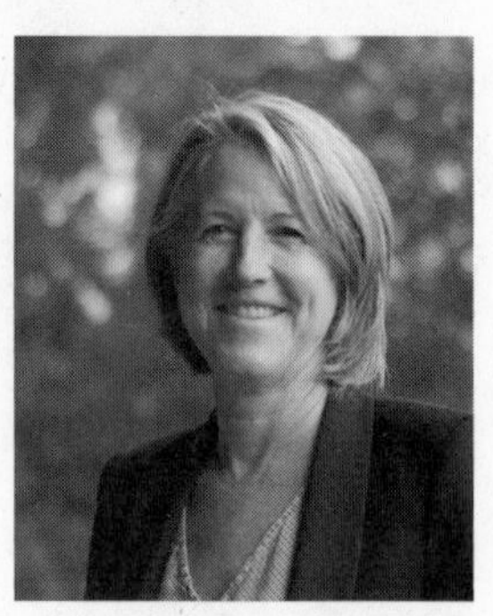
KYAWT THIRI NYUNT

Vincanne Adams, PhD, is a professor and vice-chair of Medical Anthropology, in the Department of Anthropology, History, and Social Medicine at the University of California, San Francisco. Dr. Adams has previously published six books on the social dynamics of health, scientific knowledge and politics, including most recently, *Markets of Sorrow, Labors of Faith: New Orleans in the Wake of Katrina* (2013), and *Metrics: What Counts in Global Health* (2016). She is currently editor for *Medical Anthropology Quarterly*, the flagship journal for the Society for Medical Anthropology of the American Anthropological Association.